Obs and Gynae

PG Focus Series

Renal Disorders in Pregnancy

Obs and Gynae
PG Focus Series
Renal Disorders in Pregnancy

Editors

Komal N Chavan

MD DNB MNAMS FCPS DGO FICOG and Diploma in Reproductive Medicine (UK-SH Germany)

Senior Consultant and Unit Chief
Department of Obstetrics and Gynaecology
VN Desai Hospital
Mumbai, Maharashtra, India

Niranjan Chavan

MD FICOG FCPS DGO DFP MICOG DICOG Diploma in Endoscopy (USA)

Professor and Unit Chief
Department of Obstetrics and Gynaecology
Lokmanya Tilak Medical College and General Hospital
Mumbai, Maharashtra, India

Co-Editors

Zaneta Dias

MBBS MS (Obs/Gynae) DNB NT Specialist-FMF UK

Post-doctoral Fellow
Centre of Excellence—Fetal Care
Amrita Institute of Health Sciences
Kochi, Kerala, India

Zeba Pathan

MBBS MS DNB Diploma in Reproductive Medicine (Germany)

Consultant
Department of Obstetrics and Gynaecology
CritiCare Asia and SRV Group of Hospitals
Mumbai, Maharashtra, India

JAYPEE

JAYPEE BROTHERS MEDICAL PUBLISHERS

The Health Sciences Publisher

New Delhi | London

Jaypee Brothers Medical Publishers (P) Ltd

Headquarters

Jaypee Brothers Medical Publishers (P) Ltd
EMCA House, 23/23-B
Ansari Road, Daryaganj
New Delhi 110 002, India
Landline: +91-11-23272143, +91-11-23272703
+91-11-23282021, +91-11-23245672
Email: jaypee@jaypeebrothers.com

Corporate Office

Jaypee Brothers Medical Publishers (P) Ltd
4838/24, Ansari Road, Daryaganj
New Delhi 110 002, India
Phone: +91-11-43574357
Fax: +91-11-43574314
Email: jaypee@jaypeebrothers.com

Overseas Office

JP Medical Ltd.
83, Victoria Street, London
SW1H 0HW (UK)
Phone: +44 20 3170 8910
Fax: +44 (0)20 3008 6180
Email: info@jpmedpub.com

Website: www.jaypeebrothers.com
Website: www.jaypeedigital.com

Obs and Gynae PG Focus Series: Renal Disorders in Pregnancy

First Edition: **2025**

ISBN: 978-93-6616-210-2

Printed in India

Preface

Renal Disorders in Pregnancy represents a unique intersection of nephrology and obstetrics, requiring an intricate balance between maternal and fetal health. This book is designed to provide residents and postgraduate students with a comprehensive guide to understanding, diagnosing, and managing renal complications during pregnancy.

Pregnancy imposes significant physiological changes on the renal system, and these adaptations can unmask latent kidney disease or exacerbate pre-existing conditions. From the challenges of managing preeclampsia and acute kidney injury to understanding rare conditions like thrombotic microangiopathies, this book aims to offer a clear and practical approach.

The content is structured to address foundational concepts, followed by in-depth discussions of specific renal disorders encountered during pregnancy. Special emphasis is placed on clinical scenarios, evidence-based management strategies, and case discussions to ensure practical applicability.

This book reflects the latest advancements in research and clinical practice, aiming to empower young clinicians with the knowledge and confidence to navigate complex cases. It is our hope that this resource will not only enhance academic understanding but also contribute to better outcomes for both mothers and their babies.

We dedicate this work to the tireless efforts of healthcare professionals who continually strive for excellence in maternal-fetal medicine.

Editors
Komal N Chavan
Niranjan Chavan

Co-Editors
Zaneta Dias
Zeba Pathan

Acknowledgments

We express our gratitude to all those who contributed to the completion of this book, *Renal Disorders in Pregnancy.* This endeavor would not have been possible without the constant support of many individuals.

We are thankful to all the authors and co-authors for sharing their expertise and commitment to producing a resource of the highest standards.

We are grateful to our mentors and colleagues, whose valuable guidance helped us form the structure and contents of this book.

Our deepest gratitude to our families and friends for their unwavering support, patience, and encouragement during the demanding phases of this project have been our greatest strength.

We acknowledge the support of Shri Jitendar P Vij (Group Chairman) and Mr Ankit Vij (Managing Director) of M/s Jaypee Brothers Medical Publishers (P) Ltd, New Delhi, India, in publishing the book and their associates, particularly Ms Chetna Malhotra (Senior Director—Professional Publishing, Marketing, and Business Development), Ms Kritika Dua (Senior Commissioning Editor), and Ms Pragati Singh and Mr Priyansh Saxena (Development Editors), who have been prompt, efficient, and most helpful.

Lastly, we hope that the postgraduate students find this book useful in their examinations and teachers for a quick revision. We also hope this book serves as a valuable resource, contributing to the betterment of patient care and surgical practice to the practicing obstetricians and gynaecologists.

Thank you all for being a part of this journey.

Contents

1

CHAPTER

Anatomical and Physiological Changes of Kidney in Pregnancy

INTRODUCTION

Following changes are seen in the structure and function of the kidneys during pregnancy:

- Increase in kidney size
- High blood flow
- Supernormal kidney function throughout pregnancy

We must understand these physiological changes and recognize the normal values and the mechanisms responsible for the changes. This will allow us to evaluate renal dysfunction during pregnancy.

RENAL CHANGES IN NORMAL PREGNANCY

Substantial structural, functional, and hemodynamic changes occur in renal system during normal pregnancy. Though well studied, they are not yet completely understood. These are:

- Increase in kidney size by up to 30%.
- Hydronephrosis, mainly secondary to ureteric mechanical obstruction, commonly seen during pregnancy. Because of the angle at which the right ureter crosses the iliac and ovarian veins during its entry to the pelvis, it is more usually afflicted.
- Renal function alters in response to hormonal fluctuations during the menstrual cycle, beginning even before pregnancy.
- In comparison to the midfollicular phase, arterial pressure and systemic vascular resistance are reduced in the midluteal phase, resulting in higher cardiac output, renal plasma flow (RPF), and glomerular filtration rate (GFR). These changes last for the entire duration of the pregnancy.
- Increase in GFR by:
  - 20% at 4-week gestation
  - 45% at 9-week gestation
  - 40% higher compared with nonpregnant women at term

The GFR declines to normal, nonpregnant levels, and 1 month after delivery. The association between RPF and GFR alters as pregnancy progresses. Early in pregnancy, RPF exceeds GFR, resulting in a slightly lower filtration fraction than in nonpregnant women. RPF falls toward nonpregnant levels as the pregnancy advances from 12-week gestation to the third trimester, whereas GFR continues to be elevated, resulting in an increased filtration fraction. RPF, GFR, and filtration fraction becomes normal 4–6 weeks after delivery.

It is useful to remember that:

$$GFR = Kf\,(\Delta P - \pi GC)$$

Where

ΔP—pneumatic pressure gradient between the glomerular capillary (GC) and Bowman's capsule,

πGC—mean oncotic pressure in the GC

Kf—glomerular ultrafiltration coefficient, the product of the surface area available for filtration and the permeability of the filtration membrane.

πGC is dependent on the afferent (πA) and efferent (πE) oncotic pressures:

$$\pi GC = (\pi A + \pi E)/2$$

The concentrations of protein increase from afferent to efferent side of GC, as they are not filtered. Thus, πE is a function of πA and the filtration fraction:

$$\pi E = \pi A/(1 - \textit{filtration fraction})$$

and

$$\textit{Filtration fraction} = GFR/RPF$$

Thus, GFR increases in the following situations:

- ↑ Kf
- ↑ ΔP
- ↓ π gc
- ↑ RPF

As RPF rises, a smaller fraction is filtered out at first, resulting in lower plasma protein concentrations and reduced filtration resistance, lowering πGC.

Studies on pregnant rat model have shown that with increasing RPF, GFR also increased during pregnancy, which was secondary to vascular volume expansion, and no changes in hydraulic or oncotic pressures. Tubuloglomerular feedback was reset to allow for higher GFR, which would normally counteract the rise in GFR.

Higher RPF, with only small contributions from decreased GC, was found to be the reason for the increased GFR in a human study that linked GFR to RPF. Later in pregnancy, when GFR remains elevated despite lower RPF, alterations in Kf are thought to play a role in the increased GFR. Renal biopsies from pregnant women and from autopsy studies suggest that glomerular enlargement may contribute to the increase in Kf.

At term, reduced πGC is mainly responsible for mediating increase in GFR by up to 41%. RPF was normal at this point, and GC was most likely lower due to hemodilution of plasma proteins caused by the significant plasma volume increase that happens during pregnancy. Finally, a 20% rise in GFR, 2 weeks after birth, was related to 50% increases in Kf or 16% increases in ΔP, or smaller changes in both.

The earlier-mentioned changes have been linked to a number of hormones and processes. Luteal phase progesterone may play a role in boosting RPF and GFR during early pregnancy, and this may continue throughout the pregnancy. Under the influence of estrogen, extrarenal sources such as the ovaries and decidua boosted renin production, the liver increased angiotensinogen production, and aldosterone levels were greater during normal pregnancy. Despite the revved-up rennin-angiotensin-aldosterone system (RAAS) during pregnancy, vasodilation takes place due to several factors. Angiotensin II refractoriness is increased by prostacyclins, mediated by progesterone and vascular endothelial growth factor (VEGF). Furthermore, because they reside in a monomeric state during normal pregnancy, angiotensin II type I (AT1) receptors are less sensitive.

Relaxin is produced by the corpus luteum, decidua, and placenta, and it increases RPF, GFR, and solute clearance in rats by afferent and efferent vasodilation. This activity is mediated by nitric oxide-dependent vasodilation being upregulated. However, contradictions were discovered in human investigations. In healthy participants, relaxin raises RPF but not GFR. Furthermore, no difference in relaxin levels was discovered between women with preeclampsia and normal pregnancies in a recent study, and no obvious link was established between relaxin levels and GFR, mean arterial pressure, RPF, or renal vascular resistance in late pregnancy. Increased RAAS activity mediates sodium retention and volume expansion. This results in a sodium retention of 900–1,000 mEq and a rise of 6–8 liters in total body water, with 4–6 liters in the extracellular compartment.

PHYSIOLOGIC CHANGES IN PREGNANCY

Renal

- Renal size and volume increases
- Glomerular size increases
- Ureteral smooth muscle hypertrophy
- Ureteral connective tissue hyperplasia
- Collecting system dilation
- Altered glomerular membrane porosity

Hemodynamics of the Renal System

- By the second trimester, GFR increases by 40–65%, and RPF increases by 50–85%
- Renal vascular resistance is reduced
- Initial reduction in filtering fraction
- Improved GFR
- Glucose and other sugars, amino acids, proteins, and water-soluble vitamins are all hyperfiltered

- Resistance to kaliuresis
- Increased urate and creatinine clearance
- Positive sodium balance

Cardiovascular

- As early as week 5 of pregnancy, there is an increase in cardiac output
- A reduction in systemic vascular resistance
- Blood pressure drops until midpregnancy, then rises

Volume Hemostasis

- Plasma osmolality was reduced by 10 mOsm/kg (nadir at 10 weeks of gestation)
- Preserving a narrow range of plasma osmolality
- At term, increased total body water by at least 6.5 L
- An increase of 40–50% in plasma volume
- Decreased plasma albumin

Acid–base Balance

- Mild respiratory alkalosis
- Serum hydrogen ion concentration reduces
- 7.42–7.44 increase in blood pH
- Partial pressure of carbon dioxide (PCO_2) levels are lower (18–22 mEq/L)
- Increased bicarbonate reabsorption

Hormonal

- Osmotic thresholds decrease for vasopressin and thirst
- Elevated metabolic clearance rate
- Antinatriuretic hormones, primarily mineralocorticoids, aldosterone, and desoxycorticosterone, are elevated in circulating levels
- Serum atrial natriuretic peptide levels rise
- Plasma rennin substrate and plasma renin activity (PRA) increases
- Renal kallikrein excretion increases

CONCLUSION

Physiology of kidney in normal pregnancy is now better understood with the recent advances. It is important for us as clinicians to be well informed about the pathogenesis of diseases that affect the kidneys, and the therapeutic approaches for better pregnancy outcome.

SUGGESTED READING

1. Cheung KL, Lafayette RA. Renal physiology of pregnancy. Adv Chronic Kidney Dis. 2013;20(3):209-14.

2 CHAPTER Renal Function Tests

INTRODUCTION

Renal function tests in pregnancy need to be integrated with gestational age as changes occur in plasma volume, glomerular filtration, and tubular reabsorption. The test values in pregnancy are lower compared to nonpregnant values. Therefore, values that are within normal level for nonpregnant patients may indicate renal dysfunction in pregnancy.

The basic investigations to assess renal function tests are:

- Uric acid
- Blood urea nitrogen (BUN)
- Serum creatinine

URIC ACID

Plasma uric acid normally drops by 25% in the first trimester and then increases in the third trimester during pregnancy. In pregnancy, plasma uric acid levels have upper normal limits of 5–5.5 mg/dL.

BLOOD UREA NITROGEN

The BUN usually drops from nonpregnant values of 12 mg/dL (4.3 mmol/L) to 9 mg/dL (3.2 mmol/L), and plasma creatinine levels drop from 0.7 mg/dL (62 mmol/L) to 0.5 mg/dL (44 mmol/L) as mentioned in **Table 1**.

TABLE 1: Renal function tests in pregnancy.

Variable	*Average values in pregnancy*
Plasma osmolality	270 mOsm/kg
Serum sodium	135 mEq/L
Serum potassium	3.8 mEq/L
Serum bicarbonate	18–20 mEq/L
Serum creatinine	0.5 mg/dL
Blood urea nitrogen	9.0 mg/dL
Uric acid	2–3 mg/dL

Source: Linheimer MD, Katz AI. Renal physiology and disease in pregnancy. In: Seldin DW, Giebisch G (Eds). The Kidney: Physiology and Pathophysiology, 3rd edition. Philadelphia: Lippincott Williams & Wilkins; 2000.

If the plasma creatinine level reaches 0.80 mg/dL (80 mmol/L) or the BUN is >14 mg/dL at any period during pregnancy, renal dysfunction should be considered and further investigation undertaken.

Blood urea levels are affected by both renal and liver function. Urea is synthesized in liver and its value depends on protein intake, metabolism, and liver function. Urea is reabsorbed by renal tubules and it depends on the hydration.

SERUM CREATININE

- The 24-hour creatinine clearance is the best clinical measurement of glomerular filtration rate (GFR).
- Creatinine clearance increases by 45% by 8 weeks of pregnancy and remains elevated throughout the second trimester.
- Value decreases in the last trimester and reaches nonpregnant state.

URINALYSIS

- Urinalysis remains unchanged in pregnancy.
- Normal kidneys should be able to concentrate urine to a specific gravity of 1.026 or higher while diluting urine to a specific gravity of <1.005.
- The concentration and specific gravity of urine are affected by posture during pregnancy. Left lateral position dilutes the urine compared to upright posture.
- The method of collection of urine is important. Midstream clean catch of urine specimen is necessary. The specimen must be collected before the pelvic examination; it may be collected by the examiner while the patient is in the dorsal lithotomy position.

Laboratory investigations include urinalysis of:

- Protein
- Glucose
- Ketones
- Specific gravity
- Sediment

Glycosuria

- Detected with a glucose oxidase-impregnated dipstick.
- In pregnancy, the most common reasons for persistent glucose in the urine are physiologic glycosuria of pregnancy and diabetes. However, the possibility of primary renal disease with renal glycosuria should be considered.

Proteinuria

- A dipstick sensitive to albumin is used in traditional proteinuria screening.

- Postural proteinuria is a benign disorder that affects 5% of healthy persons. It can be ruled out by comparing protein levels in the first voided urine with a specimen obtained after the lady had been upright for many hours.
- Protein false-positive results can be caused by concentrated urine, a high number of white blood cells in the urine, or epithelial cells in vaginal secretions.
- Transient proteinuria can also be caused by fever, stress, or exercise.
- Proteinuria in pregnancy should be assessed using a 24-hour urine sample and not deemed pathogenic until it reaches 300–500 mg in 24 hours.
- >3–3.5 g/24 hours is indicative of nephritic syndrome.
- When determining the relevance of proteinuria in pregnancy, keep in mind that an increase in protein excretion with increasing gestation in a known case of renal illness does not always signal severe disease progression.

Sediments

- Requires a fresh specimen, ideally the first voided morning specimen.
- Renal casts consist of cells from renal parenchyma.
- Leukocyte casts are associated in infections or inflammatory processes.
- Erythrocyte casts in glomerular disease
- Fatty casts in nephrosis
- White blood cells, casts, and pyuria may be present as reaction inflammation of the glomeruli or kidney substance.
- Pyuria in the absence of casts may be due to infection anywhere in the genitourinary tract. Finally, the nephritic syndrome is characterized by the presence of doubly refractile fat bodies (Maltese crosses) which are visible only under polarized light.

The role of renal biopsy in pregnancy is controversial and maybe potentially dangerous.

CONCLUSION

Pregnancy induces profound physiological changes in renal function to meet the increased metabolic demands of the mother and fetus. These adaptations include increased renal blood flow, glomerular filtration rate (GFR), and altered tubular handling of electrolytes and solutes. Consequently, the interpretation of renal function tests in pregnancy requires an understanding of these normal physiological changes.

Tests such as serum creatinine, blood urea nitrogen (BUN), and urinalysis often reflect values lower than those in nonpregnant individuals due to enhanced renal clearance. Proteinuria, while a hallmark of renal pathology, may also increase slightly in normal pregnancy but should not exceed pathological thresholds. Advanced biomarkers and imaging techniques offer promising tools for evaluating renal function more precisely in pregnant patients.

Awareness of these physiological changes and their impact on laboratory values is crucial for differentiating normal pregnancy adaptations from pathological conditions like preeclampsia, acute kidney injury (AKI), or chronic kidney disease (CKD). By integrating clinical context with laboratory data, healthcare providers can optimize the diagnosis and management of renal complications in pregnancy.

SUGGESTED READING

1. Cohen HT, Spiegel DM. Air-exposed urine dipsticks give false-positive results for glucose and false-negative results for blood. J Clin Pathol. 1991;96:398-400.
2. Linheimer MD, Katz AI. Renal physiology and disease in pregnancy. In: Seldin DW, Giebisch G (Eds). The Kidney: Physiology and Pathophysiology, 3rd edition. Philadelphia: Lippincott Williams & Wilkins; 2000.

3

CHAPTER

Urinary Tract Infection in Pregnancy

INTRODUCTION

Urinary tract infection is a common ailment in pregnancy. It can be either symptomatic or asymptomatic, making it difficult to diagnose. It is an area of concern for an obstetrician, as it affects the maternal and perinatal morbidity and mortality.

Normal urine is sterile, but practically, it is difficult to collect as it gets contaminated in the distal urethra. Logarithmic bacterial concentration of 10^4–10^5/mL is usually seen in infected urine. Conventionally, 10^5/mL counts were considered significant, where <1% corresponded to contamination. Bacterial counts of >10^4/mL can also be considered significant, but higher percentage of samples will be contaminated. Relatively, if a single uropathogenic strain (or one with only moderate contamination) is identified can a diagnosis be made.

It is necessary to minimize contamination to reach accurate diagnosis. Sterile suprapubic catheterization is gold standard for collection of uncontaminated urine. Collection using a sterile catheter also reduces the risk of contamination. But these methods are practically not convenient. Random urine samples have proven to be of limited use. Therefore, for all practical purposes, collection of midstream sample of urine after decontamination of meatus gives satisfactory results.

CLASSIFICATION

- *Asymptomatic bacteriuria*: Persistent colonization of the urinary tract by significant numbers of bacteria in women without urinary symptoms.
- *Acute cystitis*: Distinguished from asymptomatic bacteriuria by the presence of symptoms such as dysuria, urgency, frequency, nocturia, hematuria, and suprapubic discomfort in afebrile women with no evidence of systemic illness.
- *Pyelonephritis*: Significant bacteriuria in the presence of systemic illness and symptoms such as flank or renal angle pain, pyrexia, rigor, nausea, and vomiting.

INCIDENCE

- In pregnancy, the overall incidence of urinary tract infection (UTI) is approximately 8%.

- According to UK studies, the rate of asymptomatic bacteriuria in pregnant women is 2–5%.
- The incidence of acute cystitis is more difficult to accurately determine, as many women are treated empirically and culture not performed.
- The incidence of pyelonephritis during pregnancy is 2%.

ETIOLOGY

The following characteristics of urine make it bacteriostatic to most commensals:

- Relatively acidic pH
- High osmolality
- High urea concentration

Free antegrade flow through the ureteral and urethral valves maintains the sterility of urine.

Physiological changes occurring in pregnancy in the urogenital tract, increasing the potential for pathogenic colonization are as follows:

- Bladder volume increases
- Detrusor tone decreases
- Progestogenic relaxation of the ureteric smooth muscle and pressure from the growing uterus cause ureteric dilatation

Because of protection from the sigmoid colon and upper rectum, the left ureter is relatively spared. Increased urine stasis, weakened ureteric valves, and vesicoureteric reflux, on the other hand, enhance bacterial colonization and ascending infection.

- Glycosuria
- Physiological aminoaciduria of pregnancy
- Fall in urine osmolality

Sexual activity is a significant risk factor.

In urine, the majority of vulval and perineal commensal bacteria, as well as gram-negative bacteria from the intestine, flourish. As a result, aerobic gram-negative bacilli from the gastrointestinal system are responsible for the majority of urinary tract infections. A distended, gravid abdomen might make hygiene difficult, exacerbating the condition.

The prevalence of infection increases with age and lower socioeconomic class. Urinary tract anomalies and preexisting maternal diseases like diabetes further increase the risk of infection.

Urethral instrumentation and catheterization can further predispose to ascending infection.

BACTERIOLOGY

- *Escherichia coli* accounts for 80–90% of infections.
- Other gram-negative bacilli, such as *Proteus mirabilis* and *Klebsiella pneumoniae*, and Enterobacteriaceae

- Coagulase negative cocci, *Staphylococcus saprophyticus*, is the second most frequently cultured uropathogen
- Other gram-positive cocci, such as group B hemolytic streptococci, though less frequent, are clinically important.

Vaginal colonization with group B streptococci has been linked to preterm rupture of membranes, labor, and delivery, as well as being a known cause of newborn sepsis. Treatment of urinary group B streptococcal infection is associated with a significant reduction in preterm, prelabor rupture of membranes, and delivery rates.

CLINICAL MANIFESTATIONS

Asymptomatic Bacteriuria

Six percent of asymptomatic pregnant women who come in for their first antenatal visit have significant bacteriuria. Asymptomatic bacteriuria that goes untreated is linked to negative maternal outcomes such as symptomatic cystitis, pyelonephritis, premature labor and delivery, and negative fetal outcomes such as prematurity, low birth weight, and increased perinatal mortality.

There is increased risk of preeclampsia, anemia, chorioamnionitis, and postpartum endometritis. Fetal risks include fetal growth restriction, stillbirth, and perinatal mortality. Screening and effective treatment significantly reduce the incidence of pyelonephritis, premature delivery, and low birth weight.

Urine microscopy and reagent strip analysis, urine-based screening tests like interleukin-8 test, rapid enzymatic test, chromogenic limulus amoebocyte lysate assay, and semi-automated urine screen are used as screening tests for asymptomatic bacteriuria. According to the Royal College of Obstetricians and Gynaecologists (RCOG), none of these approach the sensitivity and specificity of urine culture and, as a result, cannot be recommended as screening techniques for asymptomatic bacteriuria during pregnancy.

Routine midstream sample of urine utilized for screening of asymptomatic bacteriuria in early pregnancy, is a Grade A recommendation of the RCOG. In women who have been diagnosed with and treated for asymptomatic bacteriuria, follow-up cultures should be done because urine may not be sterile throughout the pregnancy.

ACUTE CYSTITIS

Acute cystitis affects about 1% of all pregnant women. This condition is distinguished from asymptomatic bacteriuria by the presence of symptoms such as dysuria, frequency, urgency, and suprapubic pain in the absence of systemic disease. Acute cystitis develops in 30% of women with asymptomatic bacteriuria during pregnancy.

The presence of nitrites in symptomatic women's urine clearly suggests severe bacteriuria. The presence of nitrite on a dipstick may be enough to trigger the start of empirical antibiotic treatment.

Women who suffer from vulvitis, vaginitis, or cervicitis as a result of herpes simplex can also present with acute cystitis symptoms. As a result, an accurate physical examination must be undertaken in addition to a thorough clinical history.

PYELONEPHRITIS

Pyelonephritis is the most dangerous type of urinary infection in pregnancy, with a prevalence of about 2%. The last two trimesters are when the majority of prenatal cases occur.

Pyelonephritis is an infection of a renal papilla that can spread to several papillae and, in rare cases, the renal cortex if left untreated. When the whole kidney is infected, pyonephrosis develops; if the capsule ruptures, a perinephric abscess can develop. Septic shock and gram-negative septicemia, both of which can lead to multiple organ failure, are significant complications.

Renal biopsy is the gold standard for diagnosing pyelonephritis, however it is impracticable in actual practice. The diagnosis is made using a combination of symptoms, a complete blood count, inflammatory markers, renal function tests, blood culture, urine culture, and sensitivity testing.

TREATMENT

Asymptomatic Bacteriuria

Treatment reduces the incidence of pyelonephritis in pregnancy and, as a result, the risks of preterm delivery and low birth weight, according to a Cochrane review.

Acute Cystitis

Most pregnant women with acute cystitis seek medical help right away. For pregnant women with symptomatic urinary infection, increasing oral fluid intake is generally recommended as a first-line treatment. This is recommended until the results of the cultures and antibiotic sensitivity tests are received. It can make symptomatic women's urine frequency and dysuria worse.

Urine alkalinizing drugs have also become popular for the treatment of urinary symptoms in women, however the benefits of such treatments have yet to be proven.

Empirical antibiotic therapy is frequently started before the findings of urine culture and sensitivity tests are available. Once the culture findings are known, it is critical to reevaluate and adapt empirical treatment. In most cases, a 7–10 days treatment of a suitable antibiotic is sufficient. The recommended antibiotic agents are listed in **Box 1**.

BOX 1: Antibiotics used in urinary tract infection (UTI) in pregnancy.

For UTI:
- Ampicillin 500 mg QID
- Amoxicillin 250 mg TID
- Cephalexin 500 mg QID
- Cefaclor 500 mg QID
- Ceftriaxone 1 g intravenous (IV)

BOX 2: Analgesia used in pregnancy.

For analgesia:
- Acetaminophen (paracetamol) 500 mg for mild pain is preferred
- Morphine in small dose for severe pain can be used

Pyelonephritis

The majority of women with pyelonephritis need to be admitted to the hospital. Before beginning treatment, blood cultures (aerobic and anaerobic) should be performed, as well as vaginal swabs and a midstream specimen of urine (MSSU) for culture. Antimicrobial therapy is started on a trial basis, usually via parenteral administration. Initially, broad-spectrum therapy is used, with the treatment spectrum narrowed as culture and sensitivity reports become available. Parenteral treatment should be continued for at least 24 hours after the woman has become afebrile. If the lady does not respond within 24–48 hours and once culture and sensitivity findings are available, it is critical to reevaluate treatment.

Renal angle discomfort affects the majority of women, and analgesia may be required. Nonsteroidal anti-inflammatory drugs (NSAIDs) should be avoided because they have been linked to fetal risks of oligohydramnios and premature ductus arteriosus closure, and maternal risks of gastric mucosal ulceration and reduced renal perfusion.

Preterm labor is greatly increased by acute pyelonephritis. Tocolysis is a common occurrence. If there is a risk of preterm labor, antenatal steroids for fetal lung maturity should be considered.

Because relapses might occur after just 7 days of treatment, antimicrobial treatment for pyelonephritis should be continued for at least 10 days.

The recommended medications and their doses in pregnancy are given in **Box 1**.

The NSAIDs should be avoided during pregnancy for analgesia, according to the Food and Drug Administration (FDA). Although opioids can be utilized, the risk of addiction (neuroadaptation) and withdrawal must be considered. **Box 2** shows analgesics to be considered for reducing pain.

CONCLUSION

Urinary tract infections (UTIs) in pregnancy are a common and significant clinical concern due to the physiological changes in the urinary tract, including ureteral dilation, increased bladder residual volume, and urinary stasis. These changes predispose pregnant individuals to UTIs, which, if untreated, can lead to severe complications such as pyelonephritis, preterm labor, and adverse neonatal outcomes.

Early detection and appropriate management are critical. Screening for asymptomatic bacteriuria (ASB) is an essential component of antenatal care, as treating ASB can significantly reduce the risk of progression to symptomatic UTI. Antibiotic therapy should be guided by culture and sensitivity, with careful consideration of drugs safe for use during pregnancy.

A multidisciplinary approach, involving regular monitoring and patient education about hygiene practices, fluid intake, and prompt reporting of symptoms, can help mitigate the risks associated with UTIs in pregnancy. Addressing these infections effectively not only ensures maternal health but also supports optimal pregnancy outcomes.

SUGGESTED READING

1. Asscher AW, Sussman M, Waters WE, Davis RH, Chick S. Urine as a medium for bacterial growth. Lancet. 1966;2:1037-41.
2. Foley ME, Farquharson R, Stronge JM. Is screening for bacteriuria in pregnancy worthwhile? Br Med J. 1987;295:270.
3. Gilstrap LC 3rd, Cunningham FG, Whalley PJ. Acute pyelonephritis in pregnancy: an anterospective study. Obstet Gynecol. 1981;57:409-13.
4. Harris RE, Gilstrap LC 3rd. Cystitis during pregnancy: a distinct clinical entity. Obstet Gynecol. 1981;57:578-80.
5. Hooten TM, Stamm WE. Diagnosis and treatment of uncomplicated urinary tract infection. Infect Dis Clin North Am. 1997;11:551-81.
6. Mikhail MS, Anyaegbunam A. Lower urinary tract dysfunction in pregnancy: a review. Obstet Gynecol Surv. 1995;50:675-83.
7. Patterson TF, Andriole VT. Bacteriuria in pregnancy. Infect Dis Clin North Am. 1987;1:807-22.
8. Ronald A. Sex and urinary tract infections. N Engl J Med. 1996;335:511-2.
9. Royal College of Obstetricians and Gynaecologists. (2012). Sepsis in Pregnancy, Bacterial (Green-top Guideline No. 64a). [online] Available from https://www.rcog.org.uk/guidance/browse-all-guidance/green-top-guidelines/sepsis-in-pregnancy-bacterial-green-top-guideline-no-64a/. [Last accessed November, 2024].
10. Stirrat GM. Pregnancy and immunity. BMJ. 1994;308:1385.

4

CHAPTER

Acute Kidney Injury in Pregnancy

INTRODUCTION

Acute kidney injury (AKI) was previously known as acute renal failure. Acute kidney injury is defined as sudden decrease in renal function which occurs in <7 days and is characterized by an increase in serum creatinine, decrease in urine output, or both.

Acute kidney injury is clinically diagnosed when urine output falls below 400 mL in 24 hours (oliguria) or <0.5 mL/kg/hour for 6 hours, along with rise in serum creatinine by >1.5 times the normal value or increase by 0.3 mg/dL from baseline value.

INCIDENCE

The reported incidence of AKI during pregnancy in developing countries such as India and Pakistan, ranged from 0.02 to 11.5%.

FACTORS RESPONSIBLE FOR DECREASE IN INCIDENCE

1. With liberalization of abortion laws, a decrease in number of septic abortions was seen.
2. Early termination of pregnancy in complicated and severe cases of preeclampsia or eclampsia along with appropriate use of blood and blood products transfusion.
3. Better management of abruptio placentae
4. Development of blood bank facilities and easy availability of blood and blood products.
5. Early detection and appropriate management of shock.

CAUSES OF ACUTE RENAL FAILURE

Prerenal

- Acute kidney injury caused by hypoperfusion of kidneys.
- Prerenal is the most common type of AKI.

Causes

- Hypovolemia
- Decreased cardiac output
- Septic shock
- Acute and massive hemorrhage

Pregnancy-specific Causes of Prerenal Acute Kidney Injury

- *Acute and massive hemorrhage:*
    - *Early pregnancy:* Abortion, ectopic pregnancy, and hydatidiform mole
    - *Late pregnancy:* Postpartum hemorrhage, placenta previa, and traumatic delivery
- *Severe dehydration:* Resulting from hyperemesis gravidarum
- *Septic shock syndrome:* Septic abortion and hypotension
- Severe preeclampsia, eclampsia, and HELLP syndrome
- Acute fatty liver of pregnancy
- *Infection*: Chorioamnionitis and pyelonephritis

Other Causes

- Mismatched blood transfusion
- Thrombotic microangiopathy
- Hemolytic uremic syndrome

Renal Acute Kidney Injury

Renal disease, disseminated intravascular coagulation (DIC), hypoperfusion, ischemia, and systemic lupus erythema with interstitial nephritis. Difference between prerenal AKI and renal AKI is shown in **Table 1**.

Postrenal (Obstructive) Acute Kidney Injury

Cholelithiasis and accidental ligature of the ureters during surgery.

Drugs

Aminoglycosides and nonsteroidal anti-inflammatory drugs (NSAIDs).

Flowchart 1 depicts causes of AKI in pregnancy in different trimesters.

ACUTE TUBULAR NECROSIS

- Most commonly seen pathology in obstetrics
- Affects the loop of Henle, especially the ascending limb and distal convoluted tubule
- Caused by mild to moderate ischemia
- Reversible

TABLE 1: Difference between prerenal acute kidney injury (AKI) and renal AKI.

	Prerenal AKI	*Renal AKI*
Urine sodium concentration	<10	>20
Urine osmolality	>500	<350
Specific gravity	>1.010	<1.010
Fractional excretion of sodium (FENa)	Decreased	Increased
Urine: Plasma creatinine ratio	>40	<20

Flowchart 1: Causes of AKI in pregnancy in different trimesters.

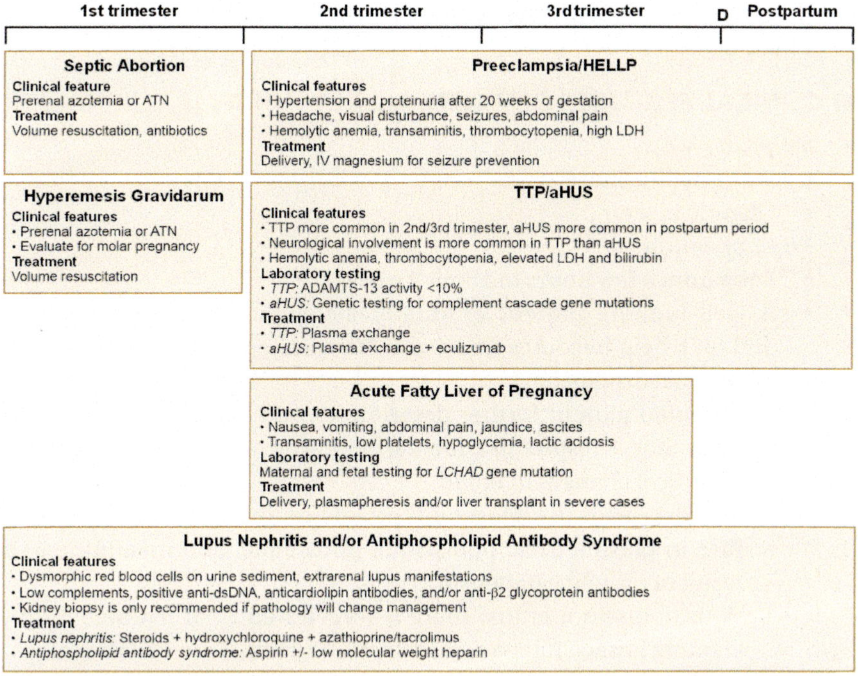

(aHUS: atypical hemolytic uremic syndrome; AKI: acute kidney injury; ATN: acute tubular necrosis; dsDNA: double-stranded deoxyribonucleic acid; LDH: lactate dehydrogenase; TTP: thrombotic thrombocytopenic purpura)

Source: Rao S, Jim B. Acute Kidney Injury in Pregnancy: The Changing Landscape for the 21st Century. Kidney Int Rep. 2018;3(2):247-57.

- Develops over 48 hours
- Grossly, the kidney becomes enlarged with pale cortex and darker medulla
- Microscopically, ischemic degeneration and necrosis of renal tubules with casts and pigments.
- Edema is seen in interstitial tissue
- If the blood supply is adequate, regeneration takes place in 1–2 weeks.

ACUTE CORTICAL NECROSIS

- Relatively uncommon
- May be seen in abruptio placentae and endotoxic shock from gram-negative bacteria
- Diffuse ischemic necrosis of cortex is seen
- Sparing of a narrow band below capsule and a part at corticomedullary junction, as they derive blood supply from other sources
- Glomerular afferent vessels are end-arteries and hence ischemic necrosis is irreversible

- Hyaline degeneration is seen microscopically
- "Rim sign" seen on contrast-enhanced computed tomography (CECT), which is diagnostic

CLINICAL FEATURES OF ACUTE KIDNEY INJURY (PRERENAL)

- *Incipient phase:*
    - Short lasting phase
    - Oliguria is seen
- *Phase of anuria:*
    - Lasts from a few hours to about 3 weeks
    - A well-looking patient gradually develops vomiting, anorexia, and diarrhea; becomes toxic, may have raised blood pressure with abdominal distension
    - If untreated patient further deteriorates and becomes drowsy, has Cheyne-Stokes respiration, mental confusion, and delirious
    - Biochemical changes in blood:
        - Anorexia leads to endogenous protein catabolism
        - Rise in plasma urea, potassium, phosphate, and creatinine as a result of protein catabolism
        - With potassium efflux, there is forceful entry of hydrogen ions, creating intracellular acidosis and thus decrease in bicarbonate
        - Rise in phosphate lowers plasma calcium
        - Rise in plasma magnesium potentiates the cardiotoxic effect of high potassium and low calcium
- *Investigations:*
    - *Blood:*
        - Leukocytosis as a marker of infection
        - Raised sodium (normal 136–145 mEq/L)
        - Raised potassium (normal 3.5–5 mEq/L)
        - Fall in bicarbonate level (normal 24–32 mEq/L) resulting in acidosis
    - Urine
    - *Electrocardiogram (ECG):*
        - Gross peak of "T" wave
        - Absence of "p" waves
        - Prolonged "QRS" complex
- *Phase of diuresis:*
    - Osmotic diuresis due to high blood urea
    - Inadequate tubular reabsorption
    - Loss of surplus fluid and electrolytes
- *Phase of recovery:*
    - Tubular epithelium regenerates
    - Function returns to normal
    - Recovery may take up to 1 year

MANAGEMENT OF ACUTE KIDNEY INJURY

Prevention

- Immediate and prompt use of adequate crystalloids, colloids, and blood at the time of acute hemorrhage such as placental abruption, placenta previa, and postpartum hemorrhage
- Termination of pregnancy in cases of severe preeclampsia/eclampsia and adequate blood transfusion, if necessary
- Early diagnosis and prompt treatment of septic shock
- Avoid using loop diuretics to treat oliguria before checking adequate blood volume and cardiac output
- Do not use vasoconstrictors to treat hypotension unless peripheral vasodilation is the only pathological cause

Treatment

- Exclude the possibility of retention of urine.
- In early incipient phase, correct hypovolemia by giving adequate blood, colloid, and crystalloids.

Anuric Phase

- *Fluid balance:*
  - In anuric phase, extrarenal elimination of water takes place through lungs (400 mL), skin (600 mL), and stool
  - Fluid loss is approximately 1,000 mL
  - Endogenous water produced is about 500 mL (water of oxidation), which is free of electrolytes
  - Thus, to maintain adequate fluid balance, 500 mL of fluid plus the total output should be administered
  - An extra 200 mL fluid is given for each degree rise in temperature above 100°F
- *Nutrition:*
  - *Calorie requirement:* 1,500–2 000 kcal/day
  - Proteins and salts are avoided
  - Adequate supply of carbohydrate prevents protein catabolism and thus minimizes urea and potassium production
  - Nutrition should consist of glucose, rice, and bread
  - Essential amino acids 0.6 g/kg is given
- *Correction of hyperkalemia:*
  - Restriction of dietary potassium
  - Use of potassium sparing diuretic
  - Glucose infusion [50 mL of 50% dextrose IV + 10 units regular insulin subcutaneous (SC)]
  - Increase carbohydrate intake

    - Calcium gluconate 10 mL of 10% infused slowly over 2–5 minutes intravenous (IV) reduces cardiotoxic effect of hyperkalemia
    - Potassium binding ion exchange resins
- *Correction of hyperphosphatemia:*
    - Restriction of dietary phosphate
    - Phosphate binding agents (calcium carbonate and calcium oxalate)
- *Metabolic acidosis:* IV bicarbonate can be given if bicarbonate <15 mmol/L, except in anuric patient
- *Hemodialysis:* It is beneficial to start early dialysis and prevent further damage

Indications

- Severe acidosis (bicarbonate, 13 mEq/L)
- Hyperkalemia (k+ >6.5 mEq/L)
- Blood urea nitrogen > 120 mg/dL or blood urea >150 mg/dL
- Clinical evidence of uremia
- Intractable volume overload
- *Prophylactic dialysis*: Urea >100 and creatinine >5 mg/dL)

In antenatal period, continuous electronic fetal monitoring should be continued during dialysis.

- At least 70 g of protein and 1.5 g of calcium should be given daily.
- Hematocrit should be >25%.
- Packed red cell transfusion may be given.
- Parenteral progesterone is given in an attempt to prevent preterm labor.

Supportive Therapy

- For control of infection, penicillin, cephalosporin, and metronidazole given
- Avoid nephrotoxic drugs
- Avoid intravascular volume overload
- Blood transfusion
- Human recombinant erythropoietin 2,000 units weekly SC
- Oral calcium, vitamin D, folic acid, and IV iron needs to be given

Phase of Diuresis

- *Fluid balance:*
    - Fluid intake = 24-hour urinary output + 500 mL
    - Oral feeding started
    - High calorie and low protein diet advised
- *Electrolyte balance:* Due to loss of surplus electrolytes, potassium, and salt supplements are given.

TABLE 2: Management of acute kidney injury (AKI) in pregnancy.

Steps	*Management*
Step 1	• History • Physical examination
Step 2	• Urine analysis • *Urine electrolytes:* Sodium, creatinine, fractional excretion of sodium (FENa) • *Urine protein excretion:* Dipstick, urine albumin-creatinine ratio (UACR), Prot/Cr, 24-hour collection • Urine eosinophils
Step 3	• Serology guided by etiology under consideration from history and clinical examination • *Example, for patients with nephritic urine sediment:* Hepatitis B and C serology, fluorescent antinuclear antibody (FANA), and antineutrophil cytoplasmic antibody (ANCA) • Antiglomerular basement antibody (anti-GBM) • Nephrotic patients FANA, human immunodeficiency virus (HIV), and hepatitis B
Step 4	• Based on the clinical assessment and above testing acute kidney injury (AKI) could be caused by: – Prerenal (functional) – Intrarenal acute tubular necrosis (ATN), glomerular and vascular disease, acute interstitial nephritis (AIN), and thrombotic microangiopathy (TMA) – Postrenal causes – Cholelithiasis and accidental ligature of the ureters during surgery
Step 5	• *Renal imaging:* Ultrasound and computerized axial tomography scan
Step 6	• Renal biopsy in rare cases of pregnancy-related AKI (PR-AKI)

Source: Acharya A. Management of acute kidney injury in pregnancy for the obstetrician. Obstet Gynecol Clin North Am. 2016;43(4):747-65.

Phase of Recovery

- Diurnal variation of specific gravity of urine is seen
- Clinical condition improves
- No fluid restriction
- Fluid intake guided by patient's thirst

Management of Postrenal Acute Kidney Injury

Accidental ureteric ligation during surgery should be treated promptly. Implantation of ureters into bladder or bilateral nephrostomy should be considered.

Stepwise management of AKI in pregnancy is explained in **Table 2**.

CONCLUSION

Acute kidney injury (AKI) in pregnancy is a multifaceted condition with significant implications for maternal and fetal health. While its incidence has decreased in developed countries due to improved obstetric care, it remains a major concern in low-resource settings.

Early diagnosis and prompt management are critical to improving outcomes, with a multidisciplinary approach being essential for addressing both obstetric and nephrological challenges. Continued research and global efforts are required to bridge the gap in care disparities and improve prognoses for affected women and their newborns.

SUGGESTED READING

1. Gopalakrishnan N, Dhanapriya J, Muthukumar P, Sakthirajan R, Dineshkumar T, Thirumurugan S, et al. Acute kidney injury in pregnancy-a single center experience. Ren Fail. 2015;37:1476-80.
2. Huang C, Chen S. Acute kidney injury during pregnancy and puerperium: a retrospective study in a single center. BMC Nephrol. 2017;18:146.
3. Mehta RL, Kellum JA, Shah SV, Molitoris BA, Ronco C, Warnock DG, et al. Acute Kidney Injury Network: report of an initiative to improve outcomes in acute kidney injury. Crit Care. 2007;11(2):R31.

5

CHAPTER

Chronic Renal Failure in Pregnancy

INTRODUCTION

Chronic renal disease can have a major impact on the outcome of pregnancy. The incidence of chronic renal disease in pregnancy varies from 2 per 10,000 women to 12 per 10,000 women. It is low because of infertility in these women, or because they are advised against pregnancy.

The National Kidney Foundation classification of chronic kidney disease (CKD) is given in **Table 1**.

Physiological changes in renal function and the markers of CKD, i.e., serum creatinine and urine protein, makes defining CKD in pregnancy difficult.

THE COCKCROFT AND GAULT FORMULA

Creatinine clearance = [[140 – age (year)] × weight (kg)]/[72 × serum Cr (mg/dL)] (Multiply by 0.85 for women)

This is inaccurate in pregnancy where this formula overestimates glomerular filtration rate (GFR) in preeclampsia and underestimates when there is a modification in the diet in these patients. Although 24-hour urine collections for inulin or creatinine clearance remain the gold standard for GFR measurement, they are impractical in pregnancy.

TABLE 1: Stages of chronic kidney disease.

Stage	*Description*	*Glomerular filtration rate (GFR)*	*Kidney function deterioration*
1	Kidney damage (protein in urine) and normal GFR	>90	50%–60%
2	Kidney damage and mild decrease in GFR	60–88	60%–70%
3	Moderate decrease in GFR	30–59	70%–77.5%
4	Severe decrease in GFR	15–29	77.5%–85%
5	Kidney failure—end-stage renal disease (dialysis or kidney transplant needed)	<15	85% and above

TABLE 2: Chronic kidney disease (CKD) definitions.

Degree of CKD	*Serum creatine level (mg/dL)*	*Creatinine clearance (mL/dL)*	*Stage of CKD*
Mild	<1.4	>70	1–2
Moderate	1.4–2.4	40–70	2–3
Severe	>2.4	<40	3–4

Source: Women's Health and Education Center. (2019). Medical Disorders and Pregnancy. [online] Available from http://www.womenshealthsection.com/content/obsmd/obsm020.php3. [Last accessed November; 2024].

The heterogeneous classification of CKD in pregnancy studies contributes to underrecognition and uncertainties around diagnosis. **Table 2** shows degree of CKD in pregnancy.

The following factors influence the pregnancy outcome in women with chronic renal disease:

- The presence of chronic hypertension
- The severity of renal impairment
- Proteinuria is present
- Pathology of the renal system.

It is critical to find out whether the patient has kidney disease early-on in pregnancy. Hematuria, proteinuria, and decreased renal function are the three most important signs to check for.

PROTEINURIA

Commercially accessible test sticks can identify it. Any positive result should be confirmed with a 24-hour urine protein concentration or a protein: creatinine ratio on a random urine sample (preferably, an early morning specimen), and protein:creatinine ratio measurements.

Persistent proteinuria (>500 mg/24 hours) before 20 weeks of gestation should ensure prompt consultation with a nephrologist. Proteinuria may increase during normal pregnancy from <150 mg/24 h to 300–500 mg/24 h. Postural proteinuria may occur which is more common near term, because of the compression of the renal veins by the enlarged uterus and because women tend to assume a more lordotic posture. **Table 3** explains measurement of proteinuria.

HEMATURIA

Because there is no indication that red blood cell (RBC) excretion rises in normal women during pregnancy, substantial hematuria (>10 RBC/mL) indicates probable renal impairment. When >85% of cells in nonpregnant women with hematuria are abnormal, there is a risk of glomerulonephritis.

TABLE 3: Measurement of proteinuria.

	*Approximate amount**	
Designation	***Concentration***	***Daily***
Trace	5 mg/dL to 20 mg/dL	
1+	30 mg/dL	<0.5 g/day
2+	100 mg/dL	0.5 g/day to 1 g/day
3+	300 mg/dL	1 g/day to 2 g/day
4+	>2,000 mg/dL	>2 g/day

*The diagnostic criterion for protein levels in PE is proteinuria of at least 300 mg of protein in a 24-hour urine collection.

Source: Semantic Scholar. (2014). Proteinuria measurement and urine-based markers for preeclampsia diagnosis Technology Opportunity Assessment. [online] Available from https://www.semanticscholar.org/paper/Proteinuria-measurement-and-urine-based-markers-for/c9f76e6c7d30b05373e89688962ab23333e824db/figure/0. [Last accessed November, 2024].

HYPERTENSION

Blood pressure (BP) drops during the first and second trimesters of a normal pregnancy, so any woman presenting with a BP of >130/80 mm Hg in the first trimester should be suspected of having a renal disease. If further testing reveals no renal disease, she is most likely suffering from essential hypertension or preeclampsia. Only 5% of pregnant women with high BP have underlying kidney damage.

RENAL FUNCTION

Early in pregnancy, failure to increase renal function is a strong indicator of the presence of underlying chronic renal disease. In people with modest renal illness, definite increases in GFR occur early in the first trimester and are maintained throughout pregnancy, whereas no rise in GFR may occur in patients whose plasma creatinine exceeds 123 μmol/L.

ENDOCRINE EFFECTS

Patients with chronic renal failure who are not on dialysis have oligomenorrhea or amenorrhea in at least 80% of cases. In 50% of these patients, menstruation returns after dialysis. It is not known whether their cycles are ovulatory. The preovulatory peak of plasma luteinizing hormone (LH) and estradiol is frequently absent, indicating a hypothalamic cause for anovulation. Indirect measures of ovulation, such as basal body temperature or vaginal cytology, indicate absent or rare ovulation, and the preovulatory peak of plasma LH and estradiol is frequently absent, indicating a hypothalamic cause for anovulation. In the absence of a preovulatory LH-follicle-stimulating hormone (FSH) surge, positive estradiol feedback is disrupted. As a result, progesterone levels do not rise in the second part of the menstrual cycle, resulting in hypermenorrhea and abnormal bleeding. These women report loss of orgasm and disinterest in sexual activity. Fertility is reduced, early abortions and fetal wastage is common in uremic women. While some women have carried babies to term while on dialysis, the majority of these women still have some kidney function. In postmenopausal women, gonadotropins are as high as in nonuremic postmenopausal women, but menopause may occur earlier in women with chronic renal failure.

An algorithm for the management of CKD in pregnancy is explained in **Flowchart 1**.

PRECONCEPTION PLANNING

Prepregnancy counseling early in the disease course is essential for women with CKD. Contraceptive options should be discussed if a delay in pregnancy is desirable, with explanation about the risks associated with pregnancy. Emphasis is given about the benefits of careful pregnancy planning. Key areas for discussion are:

- Optimizing modifiable factors such as BP and control of primary renal disease
- Implementation of change in drug therapy
- Making decisions about when to conceive
- Creating a comprehensive pregnancy management plan
- Women with inheritable renal illness should be offered genetic counseling. Single embryo transfer should be recommended to women undergoing in vitro fertilization.
- Folic acid supplementation is advised before conception and during the first trimester. Dialyzed women, on the other hand, may require 3–5 mg/day due to dialysis losses.

Pregnant women with CKD benefit from a multidisciplinary strategy that includes:

- Obstetricians
- Obstetric physicians/nephrologists
- Anesthetists
- Dietician
- Midwifery input.

Majority of women might have uncomplicated pregnancies and excellent outcomes, but require frequent antenatal follow-up to monitor maternal renal function and BP, and fetal growth and well-being.

They should be seen as early as possible in pregnancy. A baseline renal profile should be completed, which includes serum urea, creatinine, electrolytes, albumin, and a complete blood count, urinalysis, and urine culture. In addition, a proteinuria test must be performed. Depending on

Flowchart 1: Management of CKD in pregnancy.

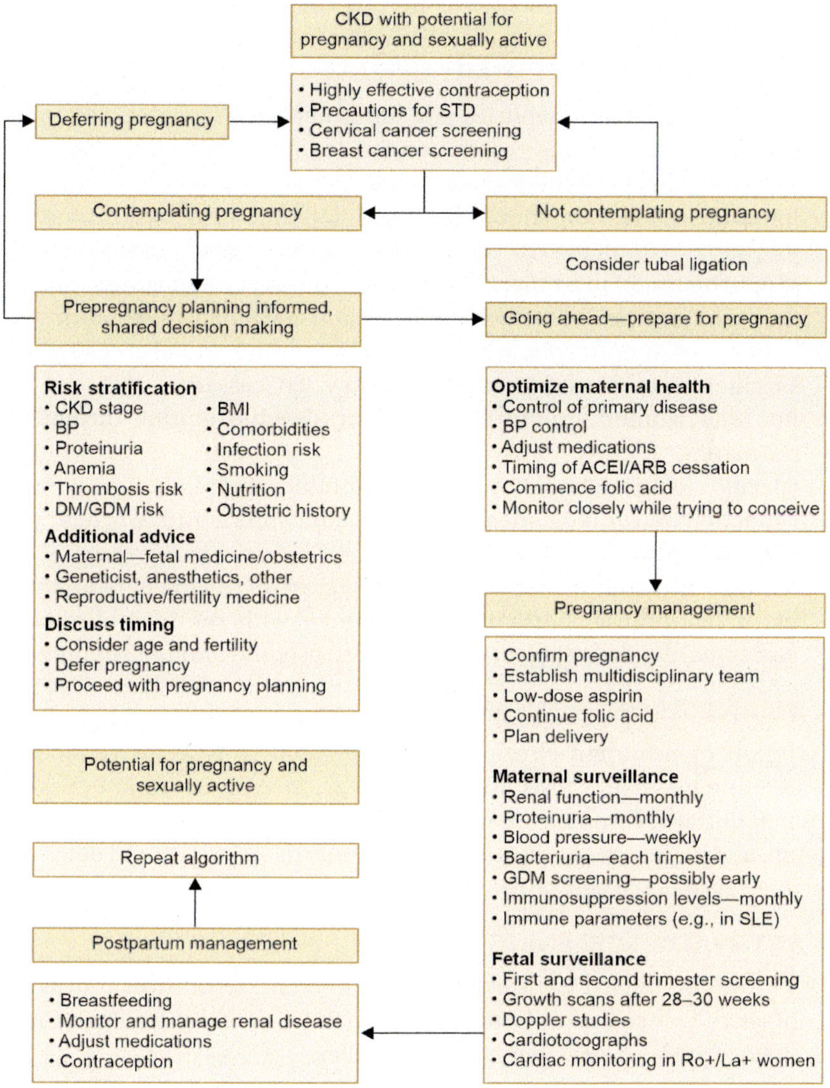

(ACEI: angiotensin-converting enzyme; ARB: angiotensin receptor blocker; BMI: body mass index; BP: blood pressure; CKD: chronic kidney disease; GDM: gestational diabetes mellitus; SLE: systemic lupus erythematosus; STD: sexually transmitted disease)

Source: Fitzpatrick A, Mohammadi F, Jesudason S. Managing pregnancy in chronic kidney disease: improving outcomes for mother and baby. Int J Womens Health. 2016;8:273-85.

the clinical circumstances, these tests should be performed every 4 weeks or more frequently.

MANAGEMENT OF PRIMARY DISEASE

- Quiescent glomerulonephritis and lupus nephritis for at least 6 months prior to conception is recommended for pregnancy with glomerulonephritis and lupus nephritis.
- Immunosuppression should be controlled and sustained throughout pregnancy to limit the risk of illness flare. Anti-Ro and anti-La antibodies should be tested in women with systemic lupus erythematosus (SLE), as they are associated with neonatal lupus and congenital heart block.
- Markers of antiphospholipid antibody syndrome are also tested, and specific management started in pregnancy, if necessary.
- Ro+/La+ women should continue hydroxychloroquine throughout pregnancy.
- Specific attention should be given to comorbid conditions.
- Diabetic control is needed during preconception and pregnancy for better outcomes.
- Routine urinalysis is mandatory, with aggressive treatment of asymptomatic bacteriuria, particularly in women with reflux nephropathy, autosomal dominant polycystic kidney disease, and immunosuppression.

DIAGNOSIS OF PREGNANCY

Excretion of β-human chorionic gonadotropin (β-hCG) is reduced in CKD. Urine pregnancy tests may be *falsely positive*. As irregular cycles and anovulation are common in advanced CKD, serial β-hCG monitoring of serum, and pelvic ultrasound are useful to confirm pregnancy and determine accurate gestational age, rather than date of last menstrual cycle.

ANTENATAL SCREENING

- Ultrasound nuchal translucency measurement, serum-free β-hCG and pregnancy-associated plasma protein A (PAPP-A) measurement are done in first trimester for screening aneuploidies.
- Free β-hCG, unconjugated estradiol, fetoprotein, and inhibin A are measured in the second trimester.
- Test validity is affected by impaired renal clearance of free β-hCG.
- α-fetoprotein levels are not affected by renal disease. It is used in screening neural tube defects.
- In early stage, CKD in pregnancy can be used to interpret risk for small-for-gestational-age (SGA) babies.
- PAPP-A is unreliable in late-stage CKD, including dialysis, and is falsely increased in heparin-treated women.
- During dialysis, unconjugated estradiol is removed.

HYPERTENSION

In hypertensive women with CKD in pregnancy, it is recommended to maintain BP <140/90 mm Hg, as per the National Institute for Health and Care Excellence (NICE) guidelines. In the Control of Hypertension in Pregnancy Study (CHIPS) trial, concerns regarding effects of lower BP on fetal growth were addressed, where tighter control of diastolic BP reduced severe maternal hypertension with no significant fetal impact.

Recommended medication for hypertension:

- Methyldopa (maximum 3 g in divided doses)
- Labetalol (maximum 1.2 g in divided doses)
- Nifedipine extended release (maximum 90 mg twice/day)
- Hydralazine (50 mg every 6 hours)

Medications not recommended for treatment of hypertension:

- Angiotensin-converting enzyme (ACE) inhibitors
- Angiotensin receptor blockers

Because of intrauterine growth restriction, renal dysplasia, oligohydramnios, and fetal mortality, ACE inhibitors, and angiotensin receptor blockers are contraindicated in pregnancy. A twofold increase in risk of congenital malformations, majorly cardiac, and central nervous system abnormalities were associated with first trimester usage. In proteinuric patients, due to antiproteinuric benefits, continuing these drugs until conception is considered acceptable.

PREECLAMPSIA PROPHYLAXIS AND DIAGNOSIS

- The NICE guidelines and ASPRE (Combined Multimarker Screening and Randomized Patient Treatment with Aspirin for Evidence-Based Pre-eclampsia Prevention) trial currently supports low-dose aspirin (150 mg/day) for women with CKD from 12 weeks until delivery.
- Calcium and vitamin D supplementation also have been evaluated as preventive strategies for preeclampsia. For the prevention of preeclampsia, the World Health Organization (WHO) recommends daily supplementation with 1.5–2 g oral elemental calcium in people who have a low dietary intake; however, vitamin D supplementation needs more research.
- Diagnosing preeclampsia in CKD is difficult.
- The manifestation of underlying renal disease is affected by pregnancy or may represent preeclampsia clinical features such as worsening hypertension and proteinuria.
- Liver enzymes and platelet count, which are nonrenal parameters, are most useful.
- In high-risk populations, such as women with CKD, soluble fms-like tyrosine kinase-1 (sFLT-1), placental growth factor, and serum placental

protein 13 may help distinguish preeclampsia from CKD and predict preeclampsia. These biomarkers are being validated in CKD patients and may have a considerable impact on future care, despite the fact that they are not readily available.

Women with CKD with superimposed preeclampsia should have their deliveries timed according to local standards for non-CKD preeclampsia, with a focus on BP control and renal function monitoring peripartum and postpartum.

ANEMIA

Reduced erythropoietin production and shorter red cell survival cause anemia in women with renal insufficiency. Oral/intravenous iron treatment is usually effective in treating this anemia. Hypertension can be caused by erythropoietin, or it might worsen preexisting hypertension. In rare circumstances where erythropoiesis stimulating medications are not thought to be safe to use, blood transfusions may be required to maintain the hematocrit.

PRETERM LABOR

Early treatment of bacterial vaginal and urinary tract infections, including asymptomatic bacteriuria, can be helpful in prevention of preterm labor. Antibiotic prophylaxis throughout pregnancy can be considered in women with recurrent urinary tract infections throughout pregnancy.

MATERNAL ACIDOSIS

Maternal pH should ideally be maintained at >7.2. Maternal acidosis will progress to fetal acidemia and may require initiation of sodium bicarbonate therapy. Electrolyte abnormalities are common in women with CKD, thus dietary counseling for a low potassium diet should be started, and binding resins can be employed.

FETAL MONITORING

A comprehensive scan of the urinary tract should be included in an anomaly scan to check for signs of hereditary disorders such as obstructive uropathy. From the 28th week of pregnancy, regular scans are recommended every 4 weeks to monitor growth and fluid volume. From 28 to 30 weeks, a Doppler assessment of the uterine, umbilical, and fetal cerebral vessels, as well as the ductus venosus, should be conducted fortnightly to provide information on fetal well-being. Depending on the gestational age, this value changes. Absent or reversed end-diastolic flow in the umbilical artery indicate increased placental vascular resistance, and occur before changes in middle cerebral artery blood flow and brain sparing, which indicate late fetal impairment. Polyhydramnios is common in pregnant women who have diabetes or have a high serum urea level. After 28 weeks, cardiotocography should be considered to assess fetal condition, especially in women who are on dialysis. Surveillance for intrauterine growth restriction or fetal compromise usually picked up by Doppler studies is imperative as this is often the primary precipitant for early delivery.

TIMING AND TYPE OF DELIVERY

Delivery should be planned at or near term if there is no maternal or fetal worsening. Obstetric indications such as preeclampsia and fetal development restriction, as well as rapidly deteriorating maternal renal function, frequently necessitate an early delivery. Obstetric concerns should be the primary factor in deciding whether or not to have a caesarean section. Following delivery, women should be seen at a postnatal combined clinic. They should continue their established care with their nephrology team.

BREASTFEEDING

Because the benefits of nursing (especially for preterm newborns) may outweigh the putative dangers of negative effects on infants, breastfeeding alternatives should be evaluated well before delivery. In addition to enalapril, captopril, and quinapril, all hypertension medicines administered antenatally are safe to breastfeed. Many immunosuppressants have little data; however, breast milk exposure is modest. Glucocorticoids with azathioprine are generally considered to be safe. Tacrolimus, cyclosporine, and mycophenolate need more data.

CONTRACEPTIVE COUNSELING

Barrier methods, hormonal methods, and intrauterine devices are the most common contraceptive alternatives for women with renal disease; however, there is limited evidence on efficacy and failure rates in women with kidney disease. Barrier techniques alone are insufficient to provide this cohort with the extremely effective contraception they demand. If the family is complete, surgical sterilization should be explored.

Oral contraceptive pills (OCPs) containing estrogen are generally contraindicated in women with cardiovascular illness, a history of thromboembolism, and smokers >35 years of age, and are only marginally contraindicated in women with hypertension, diabetes mellitus, or SLE. It is preferable to use a low-dose OCP. Other contraceptive techniques are more appropriate in women with hypertension, given the availability of safer alternatives. Progesterone-only contraceptives, such as the progesterone-only OCP, subdermal implants or intrauterine devices, and injectable medroxyprogesterone, may be an effective and safer choice. Desogestrel-containing pills have a longer window of action than other options for progesterone-only OCPs. Amenorrhea, which may help with iron deficiency anemia treatment, is one of the potential benefits of progesterone-only contraceptives. Although some have raised concerns about efficacy in immunocompromised women, nonhormonal (copper) intrauterine devices alleviate some of the limitations of hormonal approaches. Nonhormonal (copper) intrauterine devices overcome some limitations of hormonal methods, although some have had concerns regarding efficacy in immunosuppressed women.

In this group, emergency contraception is probably safe. Medical abortion using mifepristone or misoprostol has been recorded in women with CKD without complications, however due to a lack of data, it should be used with caution.

POSTPARTUM CARE

The physiological alterations take longer than 3 months to dissipate. During this time, BP, renal function, fluid balance, and pharmacological treatment should be monitored. Women who have new-onset proteinuria as a result of preeclampsia should be monitored until the proteinuria goes away or a diagnosis of renal illness is obtained.

CONCLUSION

Even in the early stages of disease, maternal CKD in pregnancy poses a variety of problems to women and doctors, with growing obstetric and perinatal risks based on disease stage and comorbidity. Preconception counseling is critical to assisting women in making educated, autonomous decisions and maximizing opportunities to change medical care to improve pregnancy outcomes. The care of these women and their newborns requires a comprehensive and specialized team approach.

SUGGESTED READING

1. Fitzpatrick A, Mohammadi F, Jesudason S. Managing pregnancy in chronic kidney disease: improving outcomes for mother and baby. Int J Womens Health. 2016;8:273-85.
2. Kapoor N, Makanjuola D, Shehata H. (2009), Management of women with chronic renal disease in pregnancy. Obstet Gynaecol. 2009;11:185-91.

CHAPTER 6

Nephrolithiasis

INTRODUCTION

The incidence of urinary stone during pregnancy ranges from 1/200 to 1/2,000 and is encountered more often in multiparous compared to primiparous women, usually in the second or third trimester.

CAUSES OF URETERIC CALCULI

- Urinary tract dilatation due to obstruction by gravid uterus
- Progesterone causes smooth muscle relaxation and reduces peristalsis in the ureter
- Pregnancy predisposes infection
- Increase in renal plasma flow and glomerular filtration rate which leads to urinary excretion of calcium, uric acid, sodium and oxalates, all lithogenic
- Urinary stasis secondary to hydronephrosis.

Physiological hydronephrosis is seen commonly on the right side. As a result of dextrorotation of the uterus, the right side is more dilated than the left, and the sigmoid colon has a protective effect over the left ureter. Dilatation starts by 6 weeks of gestation and resolves by 6 weeks postpartum.

CLINICAL PRESENTATION

Tenderness, hematuria, and fever, as well as colicky or dull aching discomfort that radiates to the lower abdomen or labial region. A tentative diagnosis can be made based on these symptoms; however, it could be mistaken as diverticulitis, appendicitis, or placental abruption.

COMPLICATIONS

Because of the possible hazards to the mother and fetus, ureteric stone management is critical during pregnancy. Preterm labor and early membrane rupture are the main dangers. Other complications are obstructive uropathy, hypertension, and higher incidence of caesarean section, gestational diabetes mellitus, recurrent abortions, and preeclampsia. These issues make accurate diagnosis of ureteric stone imperative.

INVESTIGATIONS

Owing to inability to use good imaging options for the diagnosis confirmation and invasive approach for the treatment, management becomes a challenge for the treating urologist.

Multidisciplinary team of urologist, obstetricians, and physicians with an individualized patient approach should be used, which moves sequentially from conservative to an invasive approach.

LABORATORY ASSESSMENT

- To check for underlying infection, a dipstick analysis of a midstream urine sample should be performed.
- An alkaline pH of >7 may indicate infection with a urea-splitting organism; a pH of <5 may indicate uric acid stone formation.
- If the nitrite dipstick is positive, a urine culture and sensitivity test should be sent to confirm infection and identify the bacteria.
- Blood should be drawn to check for anemia, kidney function, and any electrolyte imbalances, such as calcium.
- Increased serum calcium should induce hyperparathyroidism testing.

IMAGING

Due to its lack of ionizing radiation, low cost, and accessibility, ultrasonography (USG) is utilized as a diagnostic test in pregnant women with suspected ureteric colic. It has a high specificity and low sensitivity which can be a problem in the management of ureteric stone during pregnancy.

Transvaginal USG helps in the detection of distal ureteral calculi obstruction and differentiates it from physiological hydronephrosis of pregnancy. In contrast to healthy pregnant hydronephrosis, the presence of hydroureter distal to the iliac vasculature implies blockage. Severe hydroureteronephrosis on the left side can also indicate a pathological cause of blockage.

Doppler US (DUS) measurement of the resistive index (RI) can be used to distinguish physiological hydronephrosis from pathologic obstruction. To avoid damaging the delicate embryo in the first trimester, exposure time should be maintained to a minimum, and sonic power should be reduced to a minimum.

Low dose CT and MRI is the second line of imaging. They are more informative and safer in pregnancy. High dose CT scan is contraindicated.

Intravenous (IV) urography delineates anatomic and functional information of renal units, but is associated with the harmful radiation exposure and is avoided.

MANAGEMENT

Expectant Management

Because up to 60–80% of patients with symptomatic ureteric stones pass their stones spontaneously without complication, most pregnant females with symptomatic ureteric stones can be handled conservatively.

Conservative treatment includes analgesics, fluids (oral or IV), antiemetics, and antibiotics if needed, and is overseen by an urologist and an obstetrician.

In pregnant women, this protocol is followed when:
- No signs of infection
- Stone size of <1 cm
- Adequate pain control with oral analgesics

During the conservative treatment of such individuals, serial USG should be performed on a regular basis.

In pregnancy, the following drugs are advised, along with their dosages:
- In the case of a UTI:
    - 500 mg ampicillin qid
    - 250 mg amoxicillin tid
    - 500 mg cephalexin qid
    - 500 mg cefaclor qid
    - IV ceftriaxone 1 g
- Nonsteroidal anti-inflammatory drugs (NSAIDs) should be avoided during pregnancy for analgesia, according to the Food and Drug Administration (FDA). Although opioids can be utilized, the risk of addiction (neuroadaptation) and withdrawal must be considered.
- Acetaminophen (paracetamol) 500 mg is suggested for analgesia in mild pain.
- For extreme pain, a tiny amount of morphine can be given.
- Antiemetics (metoclopramide 5–10 mg orally before eating) and antacids (pantoprazole 20/40 mg) are both safe during pregnancy.
- If the patient is dehydrated, IV fluids can be used sparingly. According to the patient's health and investigations, normal saline, or different IV fluids can be given.

Medical Expulsive Therapy

When conservative treatment fails, medical expulsive therapy (MET) with alpha-blockers and calcium channel blockers, classified as Category B drugs in pregnancy is used as illustrated in **Flowchart 1**.

Both alpha-blockers and calcium channel blockers stop the ureter's peristaltic action, which helps stones pass. They may also aid in the reduction of colic episodes, analgesic needs, and hospitalizations.

Indications for Intervention

- When conservative treatment fails
- Progression of unresolved symptoms
- Hydronephrosis, urethritis, sepsis, solitary kidney obstruction, bilateral obstruction, and progressive renal impairment
- Inadequate urological care and equipment

Flowchart 1: Management of pregnant female with suspected ureteric colic.

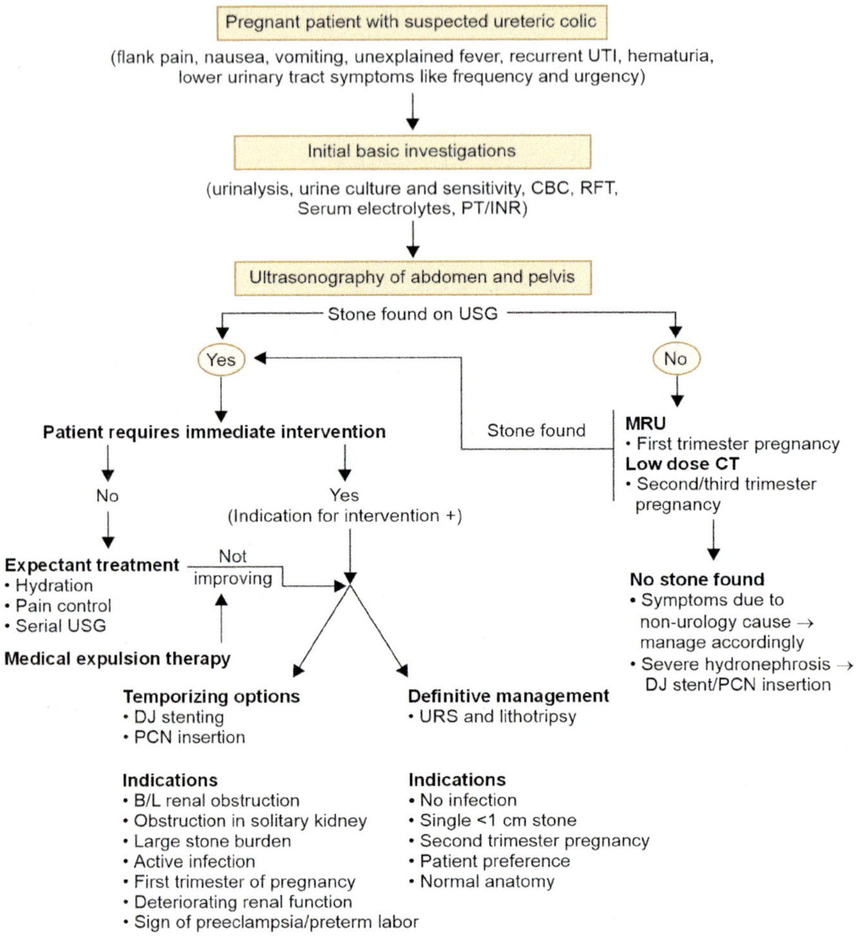

(CBC: complete blood count; DJ: double J; INR: international normalized ratio; MRU: magnetic resonance urography; PCN: percutaneous nephrostomy; PT: prothrombin time; RFT: renal function test; URS: ureteroscopy; USG: ultrasonography; UTI: urinary tract infection)

Source: Thakur APS, Sharma V, Ramasamy V, Choudhary A, Patel P, Singh S, et al. Management of ureteric stones in pregnancy: A review. Afr J Urol. 2020;26:60.

Preeclampsia and preterm labor are examples of pregnancy complications. The second trimester is the preferred period for nonobstetrical surgery, as the risk of miscarriages in the first trimester and preterm labor in the third trimester is avoided.

Approximately 20–30% of pregnant women with ureteral calculi will require active therapy at some point. Temporary drainage and definitive stone management are two types of active treatment.

Temporizing Options

Percutaneous nephrostomy (PCN) drainage or a double J (DJ) ureteral stent can be used to provide temporary drainage.

Stage of pregnancy, patient preference, and tolerability should be considered.

Stent

Ureteral stents can be placed under local anesthesia or IV sedation with ultrasound guidance. Due to the increased incidence of encrustation caused by metabolic changes in urine chemistry that occur during pregnancy, such as hypercalciuria and hyperuricosuria, it must be exchanged every 4–6 weeks. Long-term stenting has been linked to an increased risk of bacteriuria, urinary tract infection (UTI), and obstruction. Antibiotics should be started as soon as a UTI with an indwelling stent is discovered.

Percutaneous Nephrostomy

Performed under local anesthesia with ultrasound guidance, has high success rate, cost effective, and is safe in pregnancy.

The most common indications for PCN are sepsis and pyonephrosis, which require rapid pus drainage and urine samples for culture. Other circumstances where PCN is recommended include renal drainage in the first trimester, a substantial stone burden, and a higher risk of premature labor.

Tube dislodgment, the requirement to carry an extra collecting bag, tube obstruction by debris, infection, bleeding, and the need for frequent adjustments are all downsides of PCN drainage. The placement of a PCN tube is technically problematic in the third trimester, hence it is reserved for pregnancies of <22 weeks.

Definitive Stone Management

Ureteroscopic Stone Removal (URS-SR)

Indications for ureteroscopy (URS) are conservative treatment failure and patient preference.

During URS, the patient's position should be retained in the lithotomy, with the right side of the abdomen slightly elevated to prevent the uterus from compressing the inferior vena cava. To reduce complications, a DJ stent should be retained after the surgery. Fetal monitoring is performed both before and after the procedure. Recommendations include use of low-dose pulsed fluoroscopy, lead shielding of the patient's pelvis, positioning of C-arm image source below the patient and image coning to encompass only the renal area, and ureteroscope path to limit or eliminate fluoroscopy exposure in pregnancy.

Infection or sepsis, aberrant anatomy, big volume/multiple stones, obstetrical problems, and limited urological, obstetric, or anesthetic resources are all contraindications to URS.

Percutaneous Nephrolithotomy

Due to the common use of the prone position and significant fluoroscopy exposure, percutaneous nephrolithotomy (PCNL) is not recommended during pregnancy. If PCNL is needed in a pregnant woman, it is best done after the baby is born.

Extracorporeal Shock Wave Lithotripsy

Because of the danger of fetal harm, extracorporeal shock wave lithotripsy (ESWL) is not recommended during pregnancy. ESWL is a noninvasive stone fragmentation procedure that is the best treatment for small stones in the kidney and upper ureter that are <1 cm in diameter. It breaks the stone with high-intensity ultrasonic pulses.

Laparoscopic/Open Surgery

Only laparoscopic/open surgery should be considered in a gravid patient with severe symptoms if all other treatments have failed; otherwise, it is best avoided. Laparoscopic surgery may be a better option in terms of hospital stay and cosmesis.

METABOLIC WORKUP

For the gravid patient with ureteric stone, a complete metabolic workup is beneficial, but it should be done only after the patient has recovered from childbirth.

CONCLUSION

During pregnancy, ureteric stone is a diagnostic and therapeutic difficulty. It raises the chance of obstetric difficulties, which increases morbidity for both mother and fetus. Magnetic resonance urography (MRU) is a second-line study in such individuals, with ultrasound remaining a mainstay of diagnostic imaging. For the vast majority of patients, conservative treatment with MET should be the first line of defense. The insertion of a PCN tube or a DJ stent may be considered depending on the clinical situation.

SUGGESTED READING

1. Meher S, Gibbons N, Dasgupta R. Renal stones in pregnancy. Obstet Med. 2014;7(3):103-10.
2. Thakur APS, Sharma V, Ramasamy V, Choudhary A, Patel P. Management of ureteric stone in pregnancy : A review. Afr J Urol. 2020;26:60.

CHAPTER 7

Renal Transplant and Pregnancy

INTRODUCTION

Pregnancy is complicated in a transplant recipient by the underlying maternal pathology, the allograft, the effect of pregnancy on the transplant, side effects of drugs, and their teratogenicity. Renal transplantation is the most common solid organ transplanted; hence it has the most obstetric experience, literature, and clinical influence. Renal transplant recipients have 30–40 pregnancies per year, with an incidence of 2–6 per 10,000 women of reproductive age. Most women have a successful pregnancy outcome. However, they suffer from higher incidences of adverse maternal and fetal outcomes, preeclampsia, fetal growth restriction, and preterm delivery. In the United States, the median adult wait time for a cadaver kidney is nearly 4 years.

PREPREGNANCY COUNSELING

Women with renal transplants should take informed decisions as well as prepare themselves for possible complications. Conception is not advised within the first year following renal transplantation when graft stability is difficult to assess and patient is on high dose immunosuppressants. The risk of acute rejection in the first year is estimated to be 10–15% and hence contraception is recommended. Medications which are teratogenic such as mycophenolate mofetil, angiotensin-converting enzyme inhibitor (ACEi), and angiotensin receptor antagonists need to be stopped in pregnancy. Mycophenolate mofetil has been associated with an increased risk of external ear malformation, cleft palate, facial malformation, and first-trimester pregnancy loss as shown in **Table 1**. Hence it can be replaced by azathioprine. The suggested "wash-out" period for mycophenolate mofetil prior to pregnancy is shortened to 3 months, allowing confirmation of graft stability. Statins, rituximab, sirolimus, and everolimus have limited evidence of safety and they should be avoided. For nonproteinuric hypertension these can be switched to alternative antihypertensives. Women with significant proteinuria may be reluctant to lose their "renal protection" for the time it takes to successfully conceive. In such cases, ACEi or angiotensin receptor antagonist may be discontinued after a positive pregnancy test. The Royal College of Obstetricians and Gynecologists recommends aspirin prophylaxis in pregnancy for women who have donated the kidney and folic acid 400 μg/day for transplant patient planning pregnancy.

EFFECTS OF RENAL TRANSPLANTATION ON PREGNANCY

Pregnancy is a state of insulin resistance and diabetogenic immunosuppressants such as calcineurin inhibitors (tacrolimus and cyclosporine) and prednisolone potentiate gestational diabetes mellitus (GDM) and new-onset diabetes. This occurs in 4–25% of renal transplant recipients.

Opportunistic infections which affect the fetus such as rubella, cytomegalovirus, toxoplasmosis, herpes simplex, and hepatitis B and C are common in immunosuppressed, pregnant kidney transplant patients.

Preeclampsia and/or fetal development restriction which lead to iatrogenic preterm delivery are more common in women receiving renal transplants. Vaginal delivery, on the other hand, is not a contraindication. With newborn admissions, women with renal transplants, especially those with compromised renal function, must be prepared for the risk of a small, ill baby.

Table 1 lists medications commonly prescribed in solid organ transplant recipients and their safety in pregnant and breastfeeding women.

EFFECT OF PREGNANCY ON THE RENAL TRANSPLANT

Preeclampsia and acute graft rejection need to be ruled out in a patient with rising creatinine. If graft rejection is suspected, a kidney biopsy should be undertaken. Transplant rejection can be treated in pregnancy with corticosteroids and optimization of tacrolimus/cyclosporine. Because most of these medicines are actively carried across the placenta, the neonate's levels are higher than the mother's. Live vaccines [Bacillus Calmette-Guérin (tuberculosis), rotavirus, live-attenuated influenza, oral polio, typhoid,

TABLE 1: Safety of different drugs in pregnancy.

Drug name	*Safety/adverse effect*
Cyclosporine	Category C for pregnancy, safe in breastfeeding
Tacrolimus	Category C for pregnancy, safe in breastfeeding
Azathioprine	Category D for pregnancy but safer than other category D drugs, safe in breastfeeding
Mycophenolate	First trimester pregnancy loss, category D for pregnancy, no adverse effects during breastfeeding
Cyclophosphamide	Category D for pregnancy (contraindicated in pregnancy), not safe during breastfeeding
Prednisone	Category C for pregnancy, safe in breastfeeding

Source: Ponticelli C, Moroni G. Fetal toxicity of immunosuppressive drugs in pregnancy. J Clin Med. 2018;7(12):552.

yellow fever, varicella, and measles, mumps, and rubella] should be avoided during the first 6 months of life for babies exposed to biologic medications in utero. **Flowchart 1** shows algorithm for prerenal and pregnancy care in kidney transplant recipients.

Flowchart 1: Algorithm for prenatal and pregnancy care in kidney transplantation recipients.

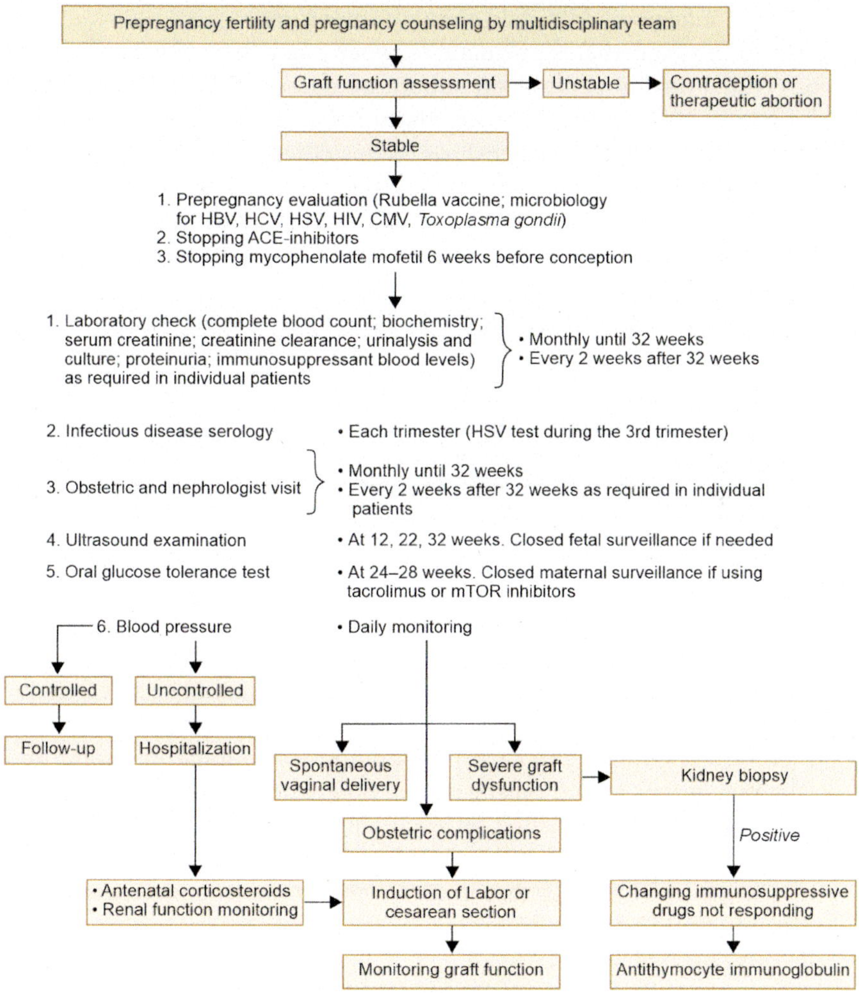

(ACE: angiotensin-converting enzyme; CMV: cytomegalovirus; HBV: hepatitis B virus; HCV: hepatitis C virus HIV: human immunodeficiency virus; HSV: hepatitis S virus; mTOR: mammalian target of rapamycin)

Source: Framarino-dei-Malatesta M. Pregnancy after kidney transplantation. In: Orlando G, Remuzzi G, Williams DF (Eds). Kidney Transplantation, Bioengineering and Regeneration. Cambridge: Academic Press; 2017.

ANTENATAL MANAGEMENT

- Renal function should be evaluated and monitored throughout pregnancy in addition to regular first trimester investigations, by a multidisciplinary team that includes an experienced obstetrician, the local transplant team, and midwifery support.
- At booking, a midstream urine sample should be submitted for culture, but isolated proteinuria in a urine sample should never be assumed to be owing to infection and should always be measured.
- Proteinuria exacerbates pregnancy's hypercoagulable state, and the risk of venous thromboembolism should be assessed. When the urinary protein to creatinine ratio is >300 mg/mmol or the albumin to creatinine ratio is >180 mg/mmol, prophylaxis is considered.
- Cytomegalovirus, human immunodeficiency virus (HIV), herpes simplex virus, and hepatitis B and C should all be tested in women. Those who have tested negative for CMV should have their titers monitored every trimester.
- Oral glucose tolerance tests should be arranged to diagnose gestational diabetes.
- Serological screening is affected because of renal excretion of β-human chorionic gonadotropin (β-hCG).
- A 12-week routine and a 20-week detailed anomaly scan should be performed. Because of the risk of growth restriction, fetal growth scans are performed at 26–28 and 32–34 weeks of pregnancy.
- Maintain a blood pressure reading of <140/90 mm Hg. Proteinuria (from a level in early pregnancy to a protein/creatinine ratio of >30 mg/mmol) or an increase in blood pressure >160/110 mm Hg should be considered suggestive of superimposed preeclampsia.
- Women on calcineurin inhibitors and/or steroids should be screened for GDM.
- Predose cyclosporine or tacrolimus blood levels must be monitored on a regular basis, with dosing during pregnancy aimed at maintaining the trough level established for each patient prior to pregnancy. Both are metabolized by cytochrome p450, and calcineurin inhibitor toxicity can be caused by drugs that inhibit cytochrome isoenzymes, such as erythromycin and clarithromycin.
- Because the demand for erythropoietin increases throughout pregnancy, doctors should consider treating iron-depleted, anemic pregnant women with erythropoietin-stimulating medications during pregnancy.
- At 30–34 weeks of pregnancy, women should be offered a multidisciplinary assessment to discuss delivery options with obstetric and transplant surgery teams. The danger of intraoperative trauma to the transplanted kidney, as well as the likelihood of a successful vaginal delivery, must be evaluated.

INTRAPARTUM MANAGEMENT

- In the absence of any obstetric complications, delivery is timed for 38–40 weeks of gestation.
- Vaginal birth is the preferred method, and prostaglandins and Syntocinon are both safe to use for cervical ripening or induction. The allograft, located in the false pelvis, does not obstruct delivery of the fetus.
- Early involvement of the urology surgical team or renal transplant surgeons is advisable when elective caesarean section is planned. The risk of trauma to the renal graft is 1–2%.
- Midline skin incision to reduce the risk of trauma to the allograft should be considered. The renal graft can also be located with ultrasound immediately prior to skin incision. Uterine incision is lower transverse.
- Stress dosage steroids should be administered to women who are on immunosuppressive dosages of steroids.
- In preeclampsia and superimposed preeclampsia, magnesium sulfate is given for both fetal and maternal indications in women with renal transplants. The loading dose of magnesium (4 g) is given but maintenance infusion levels are halved in those with significant renal impairment and/or oliguria.

POSTPARTUM CARE

- Ergometrine-containing agents are used in the management of postpartum hemorrhage but should be avoided in hypertensives.
- Oxytocin and prostaglandins (e.g., misoprostol and carboprost) in women with renal impairment are not contraindicated.
- Blood pressure should be stable and lower than 140/90 mm Hg. Women who need continuous hypertension treatment can have their medications rationalized, and the three to four times daily dosing that was required during pregnancy can be reduced to once or twice daily dosing.
- Make an appointment with the renal transplant team for a follow-up appointment. The time of this consultation should be tailored to the pregnancy's progress and the transplant function's stability.

CONTRACEPTION

Progesterone-only pill (desogestrel preparations), the Mirena intrauterine system and the progesterone implant (Nexplanon) are best suited for renal transplant patients.

CONCLUSION

Renal transplant restores fertility, but pregnancy requires careful planning. There should be an joint efforts by primary care physicians and nephrologists to include the discussion of menstrual and reproductive issues in women with renal transplant. This will enable pregnancy planning and help parents make an informed decision. A multidisciplinary approach by the transplant nephrologist and maternal-fetal medicine is essential throughout pregnancy and can result in good outcomes for mother and infant.

SUGGESTED READING

1. DC Dutta's Textbook of Obstetrics. J South Asian Feder Obs Gynae 2023; 15 (3):375
2. Shah S, Venkatesan RL, Gupta A,Sanghavi MK, Welge J, Johansen R, et al. Pregnancy outcomes in women with kidney transplant: Meta-analysis and systematic review. BMC Nephrol. 2019;20:24.
3. Wiles KS, Harding KR. Solid organ transplantation in pregnancy. Obstet Gynaecol. 2016;18:189-97.

8

CHAPTER

Glomerular Diseases in Pregnancy

INTRODUCTION

Pregnancy in young women with glomerular disease provokes anxiety to nephrologists due to lack of literature to provide the necessary care. Even the method of diagnosis, which may include a biopsy, might cause anxiety for the treating physician, especially given the necessity to rule out preeclampsia, which frequently coexists and compromises the procedure's safety.

GLOMERULONEPHRITIS

The sudden development of red blood cells and red blood cell casts in the urine is a symptom of acute glomerulonephritis (GN) (the acute nephritic syndrome). Renal function deteriorates, resulting in edema and hypertension due to salt and water retention. Creatinine clearance decreases as blood urea nitrogen and creatinine levels rise. Proteinuria is prevalent, but it is usually under 3.5 g per 24 hours.

Poststreptococcal GN, lupus GN, membranoproliferative GN, and Goodpasture's syndrome are all renal disorders that manifest as acute GN.

Laboratory investigations include:

- Antinuclear antibody examination
- Urine microscopy
- Creatinine clearance
- 24-hour urinary protein collection
- Serum immunoglobulin A (IgA) and complement measurements
- Streptozyme assay and antistreptolysin O titers

Management

- Control of hypertension
- Electrolyte balance
- Control of edema
- Uremia may require renal dialysis as they do not respond to conservative measures

Chronic GN is characterized by gradual loss of renal function, proteinuria, and shrinking renal size as a result of primary or secondary glomerular illness that has not resolved or responded to treatment. End-stage renal failure develops over time, necessitating hemodialysis. Immunosuppression may be necessary if underlying GN is suspected. During pregnancy, glomerular disorders may flare up or worsen dramatically. There is limited disease-specific data available to guide pregnancy counseling, with the exception of lupus nephritis and perhaps antineutrophil cytoplasmic antibody-associated vasculitis.

SYSTEMIC LUPUS ERYTHEMATOSUS

Overproduction of circulating autoantibodies to a wide range of antigens, particularly nuclear antigens, is linked to this syndrome. As in lupus GN, they harm tissue directly or indirectly by generating antigen-antibody immune complexes.

It primarily affects young women, and pregnancy raises the risk of a disease flare during either trimester or the first few weeks after delivery.

Factors that influence pregnancy outcomes include fetal or neonatal death, birth before 36 weeks due to placental insufficiency, hypertension or preeclampsia, small for gestational age neonates (below the fifth percentile), and maternal renal flares in women with lupus nephritis, which include severity of preexisting disease, non-white ethnicity, presence of anticardiolipin antibody or lupus anticoagulant.

Women with a history of lupus nephritis and a preserved glomerular filtration rate (GFR) had a higher risk of premature delivery and preeclampsia than women without renal impairment.

During pregnancy, lupus activity and renal function are assessed at each visit. Women with new or worsening clinical symptoms, those with serologically active disease, women who have recently changed treatments, and any woman who is clinically concerned should be monitored more closely. Antiphospholipid antibodies are seen in as much as one-quarter of systemic lupus erythematosus (SLE) pregnancies. Antiphospholipid syndrome (APS) has been linked to fetal loss and an increased risk of preeclampsia. Screening is indicated during the initial prenatal examination in women with SLE to see if these antibodies are present.

During pregnancy, anticoagulation with either unfractionated heparin or low-molecular-weight heparin is the basis of APS treatment. Pregnancy increases the risk of thrombotic events, both because of the hypercoagulable state of pregnancy and because of the obstructed venous return caused by the larger uterus. Furthermore, women with glomerular disease may have deteriorating proteinuria and frequently reach nephrotic-range readings, which have been linked to a higher risk of thrombotic events. Anticoagulation is therefore recommended for all patients with SLE who have antiphospholipid antibodies and a history of thrombotic event(s), as well as those who do not have a history of thrombotic event(s) but meet obstetric criteria for APS, such as three or more pregnancy losses or a late pregnancy loss.

SJÖGREN'S SYNDROME

Women who have anti-Ro/anti-Sjögren's-syndrome-related antigen A (SSA) antibodies should be warned about the danger of fetal heart block caused by placental transfer of immunoglobulin (Ig), which can lead to endocardial fibroelastosis. All women with suspected fetal dysrhythmia or myocarditis, especially those with anti-Ro/SSA and/or anti-La/SSB antibodies, should have fetal echocardiography, according to the European League Against Rheumatism guidelines.

DIABETIC NEPHROPATHY

Diabetic nephropathy causes complications in 4–10% of pregnancies in diabetic mothers. Diabetic nephropathy is characterized by glomerulosclerosis, which can be diffuse or nodular. Heavy proteinuria, azotemia, and hypertension are all symptoms. The specific cause is uncertain; however, it has been linked to glycemic control, hypertension, an increase in GFR, or an increase in protein consumption and excretion, all of which are influenced by pregnancy. Prior to conception, blood glucose, blood pressure, and proteinuria should all be optimized for a better pregnancy result.

NEPHROTIC SYNDROME

Nephrotic syndrome is characterized by edema, hypoalbuminemia, hypercoagulability, and hyperlipidemia and is caused by primary glomerular disease. Peripheral edema is common in healthy pregnant women, but it can be severe in those who have nephrotic syndrome. Normal pregnancy causes a drop in serum albumin levels, which might lead to severe hypoalbuminemia.

Compression stockings, avoiding prolonged standing and high-sodium diets are examples of conservative management. When conservative methods fail, loop diuretics are used to treat severe edema, and supportive albumin infusions have been documented in case reports of women with severe nephrosis.

Severe hypoalbuminemia (albumin 25 g/L) in nephrotic syndrome is linked to an increased risk of venous thromboembolic illness, and pregnancy is a prothrombotic state. However, no evidence exists to advise the use of anticoagulation in this patient population. In women with proteinuria >5 g/day, the National Institute for Health and Care Excellence recommendations for the care of pregnant women with diabetes prescribe venous thromboembolism prophylaxis. Thromboprophylaxis should be given to women with severe proteinuria and serum albumin levels of 20–25 g/L throughout pregnancy, but anticoagulation should also be considered in those with less severe nephrotic syndrome and additional risk factors, such as obesity, immobility (including prescribed bed rest), or membranous nephropathy. In pregnancy, the anticoagulant of choice is subcutaneous low molecular weight heparin. Warfarin crosses the placenta, causing skeletal deformities if given early in pregnancy and problems with the central nervous system if given later. Thromboprophylaxis should be held prior to anticipated birth and resumed as soon as possible postpartum. The postpartum period poses a particularly significant risk of thrombosis; hence, anticoagulation during this period should not be overlooked and should be continued for at least 6 weeks.

Pregnancy alters lipid profiles, resulting in large increases in total cholesterol (43%) and low-density lipoprotein (36%), as well as a 2.7-fold rise in serum triglycerides. Hyperlipidemia is another prevalent nephrotic syndrome consequence. Statins have long been thought to be teratogenic and are classified as the Food and Drug Administration (FDA) pregnancy category X. Although emerging data suggests that statins may be safe in pregnancy, they are not yet widely acknowledged. The usage of fibrates, ezetimibe, and niacin is contentious. The only class of medications that is obviously safe is bile acid sequestrants. Given the absence of data regarding medicines used in pregnancy, hyperlipidemia linked with nephrotic syndrome is often not treated.

APPROACH TO DIAGNOSIS

Kidney Biopsy

Abrupt decline in renal function, de novo nephrotic syndrome, and/or suspicion of GN are all reasons for a renal biopsy. As the pregnancy advances, prone placement for a biopsy may become impossible, necessitating lateral decubitus or sitting orientation. This scenario is frequently averted, as the hazards often outweigh the advantages of establishing a diagnosis after ~30–32 weeks of gestation. Management of suspected glomerular disease in pregnancy is explained in **Flowchart 1**.

Biomarkers

There are currently no other established indicators for use in pregnancy besides serology and complement levels. Case studies have only described M-type phospholipase A2 receptor (PLA2R) in membranous nephropathy and soluble urokinase plasminogen activator receptor (suPAR) in focal segmental glomerulosclerosis. In an ideal world, this vulnerable patient population would not be left out of future studies.

APPROACH TO MANAGEMENT

Due to a dearth of data in other primary glomerular diseases, management principles, urine protein treatment, and blood pressure optimization are extrapolated from data in lupus nephritis and diabetic nephropathy as explained in **Flowchart 2**.

Flowchart 1: Management of suspected glomerular disease in pregnancy.

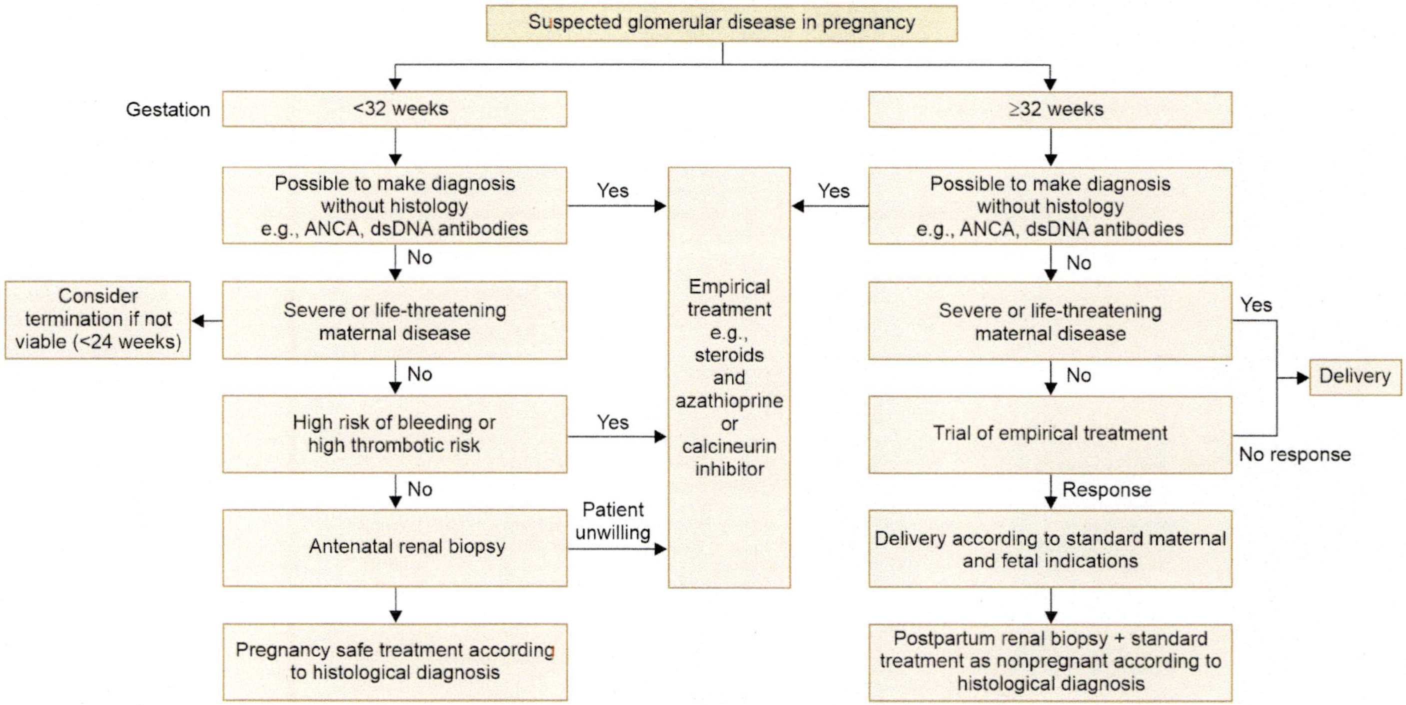

(ANCA: antineutrophil cytoplasmic antibody; dsDNA: double-stranded deoxyribonucleic acid)

Source: Hladunewich MA, Bramham K, Jim B, Maynard S. Managing glomerular disease in pregnancy. Nephrol Dial Transplant. 2017;32(suppl 1):i48-56.

Flowchart 2: Management of pregnancy with glomerular disease.

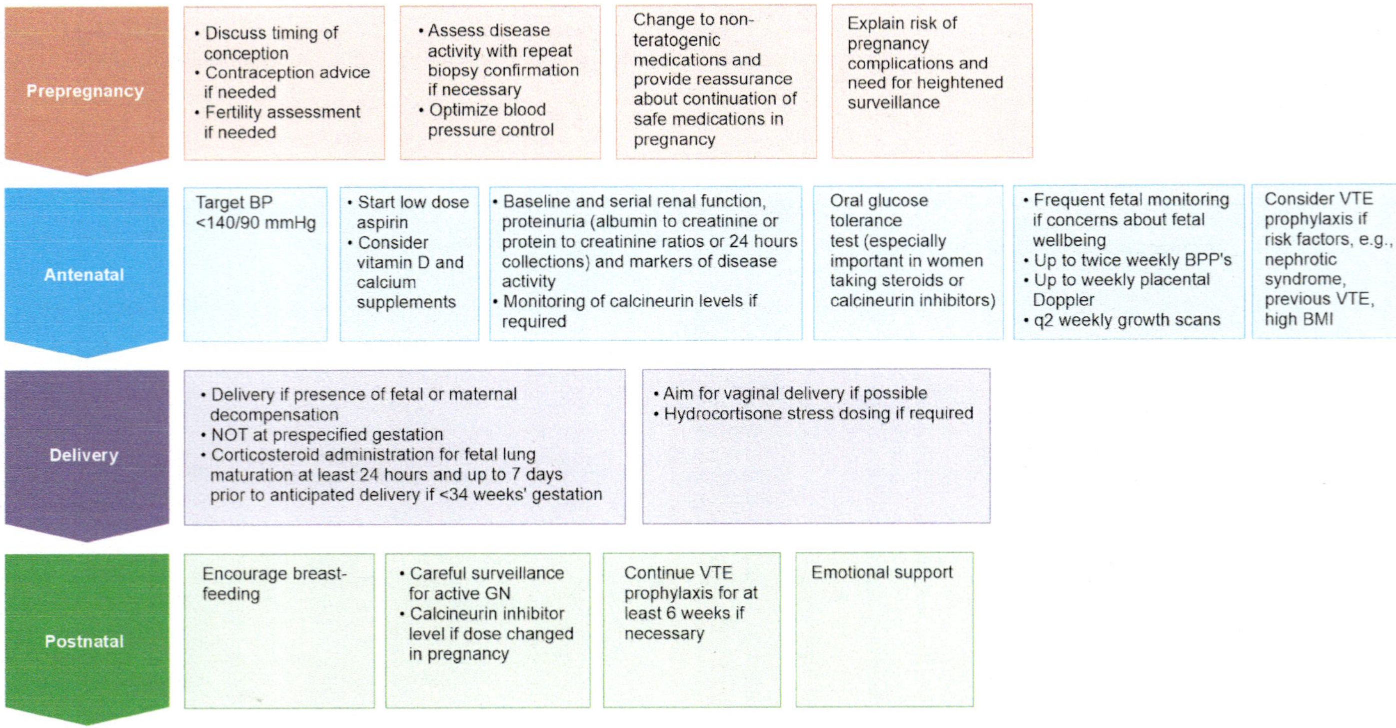

(BMI: body mass index; BP: blood pressure; BPP: biophysical profile; GN: glomerulonephritis; VTE: venous thromboembolism)

Source: Blom K, Odutayo A, Bramham K, Hladunewich MA. Pregnancy and Glomerular Disease: A Systematic Review of the Literature with Management Guidelines. Clin J Am Soc Nephrol. 2017;12(11):1862-72.

PREPREGNANCY CARE

Contraception

Estrogen-containing contraception is not recommended for women with vascular illness and should be used with caution in young women with hypertension and chronic kidney disease (CKD) because it increases the risk of thrombosis and hypertension exacerbation. Estrogen can aggravate proteinuria that has already developed, presumably due to stimulation of the renin–angiotensin system (RAS). As a result, progesterone-only preparations such as depot injections, progesterone pills, and an intrauterine device are employed. Barrier contraception is not suggested as a sole form of birth control since it is less reliable.

Fertility

Renal dysfunction produces hormonal imbalances, and drug therapy side effects such as fatigue, depressive symptoms, and a change in body image have an impact on fertility. Assisted conception is more commonly used in women with GN, but cyclophosphamide should be used with caution because there is a direct link between ovarian damage and the prescribed dose, duration, and route of administration of this medication, with oral cyclophosphamide inducing a more sustained amenorrhea than intravenous administration.

Disease Optimization

In women with lupus nephritis and vasculitis, clinical remission before pregnancy improves maternal and fetal outcomes. Treatment with pregnancy-safe immunosuppression to achieve remission for at least 3–6 months before attempting a pregnancy is a reasonable option. In individuals who do not have immunologic therapeutic alternatives, urinary protein control with RAS inhibitors is the basis of therapy. Renin–angiotensin–aldosterone system (RAAS) blockage was used to lower proteinuria prior to conception and was stopped at the time of conception, in addition to glycemic control. As a result, with appropriate counseling and cautious pregnancy surveillance, this method may be used in women who do not have immunological therapy choices.

ANTENATAL CARE

Immunosuppression

Prednisone is generally regarded safe during pregnancy, and the benefits of continuing to take it usually outweigh any risks. Prednisone is converted to inactive cortisone by placental 11β-hydroxysteroid dehydrogenase type 2; unlike dexamethasone, which is not inactivated and exposes the fetus to approximately 30% of the maternal dose. Premature rupture of membranes, gestational diabetes, weight gain, hypertension, osteoporosis, cataracts, infection, and mood disorders have all been linked to high doses of prednisone. For women who have been taking the equivalent of prednisone 20 mg or more for >3 weeks, glucocorticoids stress doses (usually hydrocortisone) are recommended during birth.

Azathioprine is used to treat illness that requires inosinate pyrophosphorylase activation to produce the metabolite 6-mercaptopurine, which is not present in the fetal liver. Calcineurin inhibitors, such as cyclosporine or tacrolimus are safe during pregnancy; however, their dose increases by 25% due to increased hepatic metabolism. Teratogenic drugs like cyclophosphamide and mycophenolate mofetil have been linked to ear, calvaria, and craniofacial anatomy, as well as limb and visceral organ abnormalities. Up to 15% of babies exposed to mycophenolate mofetil during the first trimester have significant congenital malformations like cleft lip and palate, micrognathia, hypertelorism, and microtia with external auditory canal atresia.

The nephrologist's role includes directing the discontinuation of medicines that may harm the fetus while also providing comfort about safe medication use both before and during pregnancy, emphasizing the importance of controlling maternal illness for optimal pregnancy outcomes.

Management of Hypertension

Preventative interventions are appropriate for all women with GN. Aspirin and calcium supplements at low doses are now considered standard of therapy. For high blood pressure, the drugs methyldopa, labetalol, hydralazine, and long-acting nifedipine are recommended as listed in **Table 1**. Despite the fact that diuretics are frequently avoided due to the theoretical risk of intravascular constriction, they can be utilized in certain women. Magnesium sulfate can be recommended to avoid eclampsia; however, it should be taken with caution in women who have kidney disease.

Delivery

To establish the diagnosis and manage these women, a collaborative effort between high-risk obstetrics and nephrology is required. A false diagnosis of preeclampsia will result in unnecessary urgent delivery and iatrogenic prematurity, whereas failure to detect superimposed preeclampsia may have severe maternal and fetal consequences.

The existence or severity of GN should not impact the mode of delivery, which should be governed by conventional obstetric practice.

POSTPARTUM CARE

During pregnancy and breastfeeding, antihypertensive and immunosuppressive medications are safe. The shift in maternal physiology,

TABLE 1: Management of hypertension in pregnancy.

Management of hypertension	• Methyldopa • Labetalol • Long-acting nifedipine • Hydralazine • Amlodipine (used in Europe, but presently limited published safety data) • Thiazide diuretics (typically avoided, but can be considered in difficult to control hypertension) • Renin–angiotensin system (RAS) blockade strictly contraindicated in pregnancy, but enalapril, captopril, and quinapril do not pass into breast milk and can be used postpartum to manage hypertension and proteinuria
Immunosuppression	• Prednisone • Intravenous (IV) methylprednisolone • Azathioprine • Calcineurin inhibitors • Rituximab (can be considered early in pregnancy, but no long-term safety data on exposed infants) • Plasmapheresis
Preeclampsia prevention	• Low-dose aspirin (75–81 mg daily) • Calcium and vitamin D supplementation (in women who may be deficient)
Nephrotic syndrome	• Low-molecular-weight heparin • Furosemide

Source: Blom K, Odutayo A, Bramham K, Hladunewich MA. Pregnancy and Glomerular Disease: A Systematic Review of the Literature with Management Guidelines. Clin J Am Soc Nephrol. 2017;12(11):1862-72.

on the other hand, necessitates an early appraisal of trough levels and dose readjustment to avoid nephrotoxicity in both the mother and, perhaps, the infant. Proteinuria can be targeted with RAS inhibition as early as the postpartum period. It is optimal to wait roughly 4–6 weeks for complete clearance of any coexisting endotheliosis in individuals whose renal biopsy has been postponed to the postpartum period, but the clinical situation will define the most appropriate timing.

It is impossible to overestimate the emotional toll that these high-risk pregnancies can have on a young woman. Screening for postpartum depression and a lack of coping skills is required, as is multidisciplinary assistance for the mother's health.

CONCLUSION

Pregnancy can be challenging for women with glomerular disease, however, it can be safe if the disease is quiescent and renal function is preserved.

Prepregnancy counseling allows women to make an informed choice about pursuing a pregnancy that is likely to be more medicalized and higher risk than the general population. With this approach (prepregnancy counseling followed by management in a multidisciplinary setting, close antenatal surveillance, and judicious use of appropriate medications), many women have successful pregnancies. Looking after women before and during these pregnancies, although sometimes is challenging and is very rewarding.

SUGGESTED READING

1. Blom K, Odutayo A, Bramham K, Hladunewich MA. Pregnancy and Glomerular Disease: A Systematic Review of the Literature with Management Guidelines. Clin J Am Soc Nephrol. 2017;12(11):1862-72.
2. Hladunewich MA, Bramham K, Jim B, Maynard S. Managing glomerular disease in pregnancy. Nephrol Dial Transplan. 2017;32(suppl_1):i48-56.
3. Mohammed RHA, Mumtaz H, Sangah AB, Shaikh SS, Nasir N, Jabeen S. Pregnancy in lupus: an updated consensus to guide best practice strategies. Egypt Rheumatol *R*ehabil. 2022;49:67.

9

CHAPTER

Renal Malignancy in Pregnancy

INTRODUCTION

The incidence of cancer diagnosed in pregnant women in developed societies is 1:1,000, common tumors being breast cancer, cervical cancer, and melanoma. Renal cell carcinoma (RCC) is rare and accounts for 3% of adult malignancies.

The presenting symptoms of RCC are:

1. Abdominal mass (88%)—may be obscured by the gravid uterus
2. Pain (50%)—hypernephrosis that accompanies pregnancy adds to the pain
3. Hematuria

   These three features form the classical triad of RCC.

Other symptoms like hypertension (18%) may mimic preeclampsia. Fever (21%), weight loss (9%), and oligemic shock from hemorrhage into the tumor (3%) can also occur.

The diagnosis is made more frequently incidentally during ultrasound examination.

EPIDEMIOLOGY

Factors associated with renal cancer are smoking, chronic diuretic use, obesity, hypertension, diabetes, and a female body mass index (BMI) >35.

Estrogen receptor gene polymorphism is hypothesized to have a role in the pathogenesis; high estrogen levels may promote malignant changes by stimulating renal cell proliferation either directly or via growth factors.

Also, normal pregnancy is associated with hyperfiltration which could play a role in the development of glomerulosclerosis. This makes the nephrons vulnerable for exposure to carcinogens.

STAGING

The tumor, node, and metastases (TNM) classification of the American Joint Committee on Cancer can be used to stage RCCs as follows:

- *Stage I:* RCCs that are 7 cm or smaller and restricted to the kidney
- *Stage II:* RCCs have grown to a size of >7 cm but are still restricted to the organ

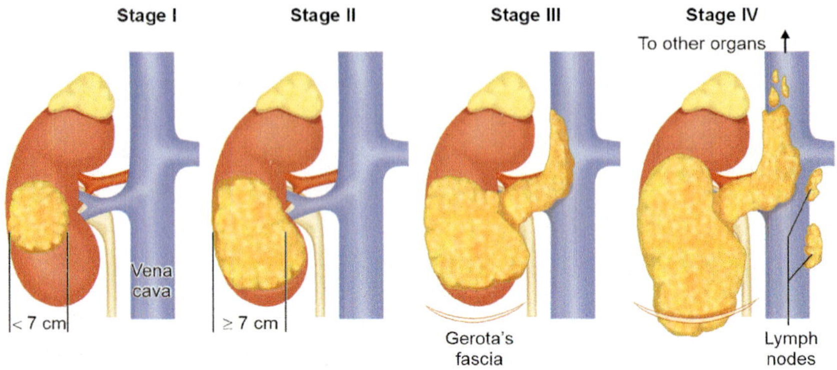

Fig. 1: Renal cell carcinoma staging.
Source: https://www.google.com/url?sa=i&url=https%3A%2F%2Fspeciality.medicaldialogues.in%2Fpercutaneous-ablation-an-effective-alternative-to-surgery-in-early-renal-cell-carcinoma&psig=AOvVaw2zW2CmQqSNAqMNhuOXLoWR&ust=1734609528758000&source=images&cd=vfe&opi=89978449&ved=0CBcQjhxqFwoTCLC689SgsYoDFQAAAAAdAAAAABAJ

- *Stage III:* Tumors have progressed to local lymph nodes, extending into the renal vein or vena cava, involving the ipsilateral adrenal gland and/or perinephric fat
- *Stage IV*: Tumors have migrated beyond the Gerota fascia to local or distant nodes, or to distant metastases

  Figure 1 shows diagrammatic representation of RCC staging.

INVESTIGATIONS AND IMAGING

In nonpregnant patients, intravenous pyelography (IVP) and abdominal CT are the modalities for evaluation. Biological effects of the ionizing radiation such as miscarriages, still birth, congenital malformation, and intrauterine growth restriction (IUGR) restrict its use in pregnancy.

- Urine sample for cytological analysis, although its sensitivity is low and false-negative results are common.
- *Abdomino-pelvic ultrasound:* Its sensitivity is 85% for renal masses >3 cm.
- *Intravenous urography:* It is not cost-effective since prenatal radiation exposure is 10–45 mGy and tiny tumors may be missed.
- *CT of the abdomen/pelvis:* This procedure exposes the uterus to 18–25 mGy and should be avoided unless there is a medical emergency. **Flowchart 1** explains approach to renal mass in pregnancy on CT scan.
- *MRI*: Investigation of choice in pregnancy. It can adequately identify, differentiate, and stage solid renal masses. However, intravenous gadolinium contrast should not be used. **Flowchart 2** shows approach to renal mass on MRI.
- *Renal radionucleotide scan:* Less radiation exposure than routine X-ray films and can determine function of the contralateral kidney and

Flowchart 1: Approach to renal mass—CT.

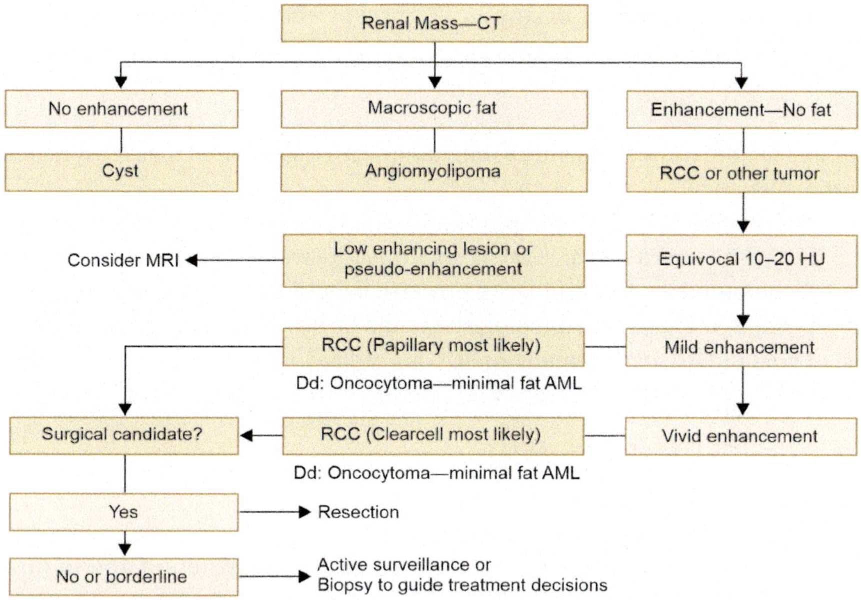

(RCC: renal cell carcinoma)

Source: Reinhard R, van der Zon-Conijn M, Smithuis R. Solid Renal Masses. The Netherlands: Radiology department of the Onze Lieve Vrouwe Gasthuis in Amsterdam, Medical Center Haaglanden-Bronovo in The Hague, Leiden University Medical Center in Leiden, and the Alrijne hospital in Leiderdorp; 2016.

Flowchart 2: Approach to renal mass—MRI.

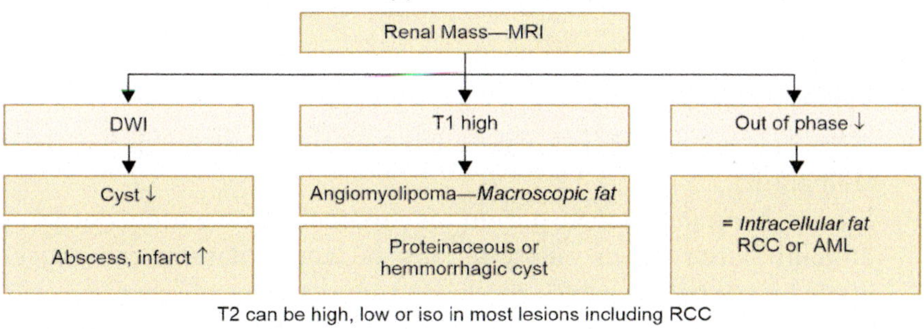

(AML: angiomyolipoma; DWI: diffusion-weighted imaging; RCC: renal cell carcinoma)

Source: Reinhard R, van der Zon-Conijn M, Smithuis R. Solid Renal Masses. The Netherlands: Radiology department of the Onze Lieve Vrouwe Gasthuis in Amsterdam, Medical Center Haaglanden-Bronovo in The Hague, Leiden University Medical Center in Leiden, and the Alrijne hospital in Leiderdorp; 2016.

intrinsic activity. Radiopharmaceuticals and contrast agents can across the placenta; hence, Doppler assessment of the contralateral kidney is preferred.

- *Biopsy:* It is not mandatory for diagnosis, as radiological studies provide sufficient findings for diagnosis. Cystoscopy and ultrasound guided fine-needle aspiration biopsy are safe and should be performed when indicated.

TREATMENT

Points to note while managing a pregnancy with a solid renal mass suspicious for malignancy:

- The obstetrician's main responsibility is to the pregnant woman, although her wishes must be considered regarding the welfare of the fetus.
- A combined team of urologists, obstetricians, radiologists, neonatologists, histopathologists and oncologists should be involved in the management.
- The standard management for RCC is a radical nephrectomy, involving the en bloc removal of the kidney and perinephric fat within Gerota's fascia.

SURGICAL MANAGEMENT

- Transperitoneal approach
- *Extraperitoneal approach:* Avoids disruption of the peritoneal cavity and theoretically may be associated with less uterine irritation and in turn fewer obstetric complications, including preterm labor.
- *Laparoscopic technique:* Reduces postoperative morbidity and pain, and allows for a faster return to normal activity levels. Injury to the pregnant uterus, as well as technical challenges caused by the growing size of the gravid uterus, should be taken into account. Furthermore, the pneumoperitoneum raises intra-abdominal pressure, reducing blood supply to the uterus by lowering maternal venous return and cardiac output.

WHEN TO OPERATE?

1. *First trimester:* Increase risk of threatened abortion, with problems of fetal prematurity.
2. *Second trimester:* Safest period, as surgical intervention becomes difficult as the uterus enlarges. Surgical manipulations can trigger uterine contractions, which can lead to spontaneous miscarriage; also, hypotension caused by blood loss during surgery can cause fetal hypoxia, which is harmful to the fetus. As a result, surgery should be postponed until the fetal lung matures.
3. If the tumor is not resectable because of development of metastases, termination of pregnancy is advised.

SYSTEMIC TREATMENT

Chemotherapy and hormonal treatment (progesterone) have been replaced with targeted therapy.

Multikinase inhibitors (sunitinib, sorafenib, axitinib, and pazopanib), mammalian target of rapamycin (mTOR) inhibitors (everolimus and temsirolimus), antiangiogenic drugs (bevacizumab), and immunological agents are the current therapy choices (high-dose interleukin 2 and recently check-point inhibitors).

The safety of these drugs during pregnancy is poorly studied with data only available from animal studies. The US Food and Drug Administration (FDA) categorizes sunitinib, sorafenib, axitinib, pazopanib,and temsirolimus as category D, while bevacizumab and everolimus are categorized C and D.

- *Chemotherapy:* Not administered during the first trimester, but can be safely given during the second and the third trimesters.
- *Hormonal therapy:* Progestogen has been abandoned as it is ineffective.
- *Curative radiotherapy:* RCC is a radioresistant tumor. It is contraindicated due to possible serious damages to the fetus.

CONCLUSION

- A renal mass identified during pregnancy can be malignant, although this is rare.
- The recommended treatment for RCC in pregnancy continues to be radical surgical excision regardless of the duration of pregnancy.
- Maternal and fetal prognosis is excellent, not different from that of nonpregnant patients with renal cancer.

SUGGESTED READING

1. Boussios S, Pavlidis N. Renal cell carcinoma in pregnancy: a rare coexistence. Clin Transl Oncol. 2014;16(2):122-7.
2. Pearson GA, Eckford SD. Renal cell carcinoma in pregnancy. J Obstet Gynecol. 2009;29(1):53-4.

10

CHAPTER

Management of Renal Disease in Pregnancy

INTRODUCTION

Multidisciplinary clinics of an obstetrician, nephrologist, urosurgeon, and specialist midwife should be involved in the management of kidney disease in pregnancy.

PREPREGNANCY

- Pregnancy planning should be individualized and partner should be involved.
- Counseling should allow for the discussion and, where possible, modification of risk factors that are reversible, such as familial conditions and medication changes.
- Disease activity should be stabilized on minimal doses of pregnancy-appropriate medications as explained in **Figure 1**.
- Blood pressure should be optimized (<140/90 mm Hg) on medications.
- Glycemic control should be ensured in women with diabetes mellitus.
- Risk of exposure to teratogenic medications should be minimized.
- Treatment plan for hyperemesis or disease exacerbation/relapse should be planned prepregnancy.
- Genetic counseling for families with a history of renal disease that may be inherited. The clinical genetics team assists with genetic diagnosis, tests family members, and discusses the likelihood of genetic diagnosis prior to implantation (PGD). The Human Fertilisation and Embryology Authority has approved PGD for autosomal dominant and recessive polycystic kidney disease, Alport syndromes, Fabry disease, and cystinosis, and some families may choose to pursue it.
- Fertility preservation should be considered for women of reproductive age who require cyclophosphamide treatment, as should early examination and treatment for infertility in these women.
- A 3-month gap before conception is recommended to allow for conversion to a pregnancy-safe alternative and maintain disease/kidney function stability.
- If in vitro fertilization (IVF) or assisted reproduction is required, women should be advised to have a single-embryo transfer.

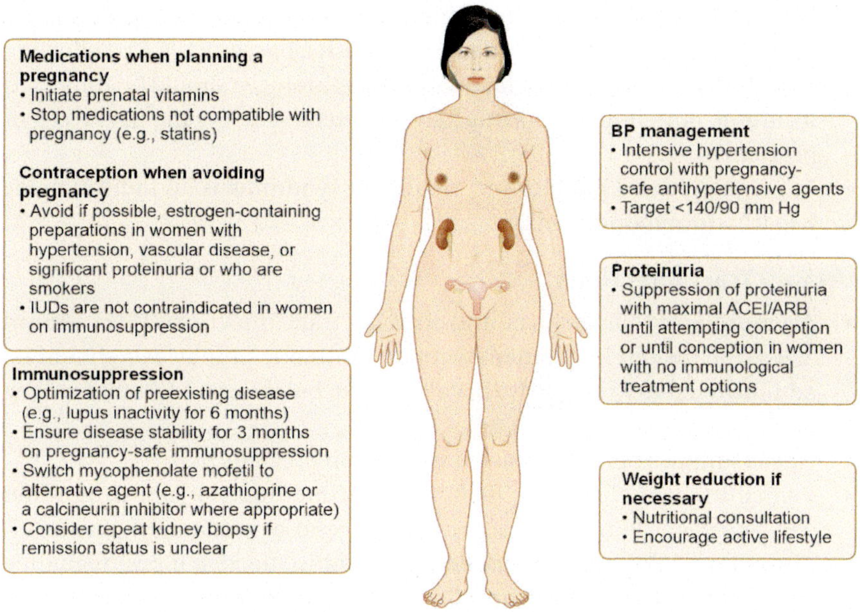

Fig. 1: Preconception optimization in women with renal disease. (ACEI: angiotensin-converting enzyme inhibitor; ARB: angiotensin receptor blocker; BP: blood pressure; IUDs: intrauterine devices)

Source: Hladunewich MA, Melamed N, Bramham K. Pregnancy across the spectrum of chronic kidney disease. Kidney Int. 2016;89(5):995-1007.

ANTENATAL

Blood Investigations

- Renal function should be examined monthly until 28 weeks, then every 2 weeks until term by creatinine clearance, blood urea nitrogen (BUN), serum creatinine level, and electrolytes, in addition to the routine antenatal care (ANC) profile of blood studies.
- Using the Modification of Diet in Renal Disease (MDRD) formula to calculate estimated glomerular filtration rate (eGFR) is not suggested during pregnancy.

Proteinuria

- Women with +1 dipstick positive proteinuria (in the absence of infection) should have their proteinuria measured. Albumin is detected preferentially by dipstick testing.
- Dehydration, exertion, illness, and alkaline urine cause false positives, while dilute urine and nonalbumin proteinuria cause false negatives.

- Urine protein and protein/creatinine ratio (PCR) should be measured accurately over a 24-hour period to establish a baseline (PCR). Following that, PCR might be used for follow-up. A nephrologist should be consulted if chronic proteinuria (>500 mg/day) is detected before the 20th week of pregnancy.
- In pregnancy and puerperium, nephrotic syndrome is an indication for heparin thromboprophylaxis.

Urinary Tract Infections

- Asymptomatic bacteriuria and urinary tract infection (UTI) should always be treated in pregnant women. Antibiotic prophylaxis should be administered to women who have recurrent bacteriuria/UTIs and kidney issues.
- Not all antimicrobials are considered safe in pregnancy.
- Penicillin, cephalosporin, fosfomycin, trimethoprim (not in the first trimester), and nitrofurantoin (not at the end of pregnancy, glucose-6-phosphate dehydrogenase deficiency, and ineffective if prepregnancy eGFR 45 mL/min/1.73 m^2) are all effective antibiotics.

Blood Pressure

- Starting in the first trimester, women with renal illness should be given low-dose aspirin as a preeclampsia prophylactic.
- Kidney donors are also offered low dose aspirin (75–150 mg) to reduce the risk of preeclampsia.
- The target blood pressure should be below 140/90 mm Hg.
- Hypertension is treated with labetalol, nifedipine, and methyldopa. Diuretics, angiotensin-converting enzyme inhibitors, and angiotensin receptor antagonists should all be avoided.

Anemia

- The most common cause of anemia in pregnancy is iron deficiency, which is estimated to affect >40% of pregnancies.
- Although oral iron is cheap and accessible, intravenous route may offer better bioavailability and tolerability in pregnancy.

Because women with chronic kidney disease (CKD) may not be able to produce enough erythropoietin during pregnancy, supplementing with synthetic erythropoietin may be necessary, even in the case of mild or moderate renal impairment.

Calcium and Vitamin D

Vitamin D supplementation is recommended for bone health, while calcimimetics and noncalcium phosphate binders should be avoided.

Immunosuppressant

- Prednisolone, azathioprine, cyclosporine, or tacrolimus, alone or in combination, do not appear to cause fetal abnormalities and should not be stopped during pregnancy; however, the safety of mycophenolate mofetil/enteric-coated mycophenolic acid, sirolimus/everolimus, or rituximab is unknown as shown in **Figure 1**.
- In pregnant and postpartum women using tacrolimus or cyclosporine, medications that interact with calcineurin inhibitor metabolism (e.g., erythromycin and clarithromycin) should be avoided.
- Because of the documented link between steroids and calcineurin inhibitors and decreased glucose metabolism, women taking these drugs should be screened for gestational diabetes.

Renal Interventions

- Renal biopsy can be conducted in the first and early second trimesters of pregnancy if a histological diagnosis will affect therapy.
- Clinicians treating women who have had kidney transplants and/or lower urological surgery should, if necessary, include the relevant surgical team in the delivery plan.
- Kidney units should collaborate with obstetric units to develop a "plan for care of women receiving or starting dialysis in pregnancy", which will be implemented when a dialysis patient becomes pregnant or a pregnant woman requires fresh dialysis.

Fetal Monitoring

- Women with kidney disease should be offered usual trisomy screening.
- If their renal function is abnormal, pretest counseling for combination screening with blood indicators should include a discussion of the possibility of a higher false-positive rate since the multiple of the median for beta-human chorionic gonadotropin may be increased.
- Noninvasive prenatal testing of cell-free fetal DNA depends upon local availability and is expensive. Fetal growth and well-being must be carefully monitored.
- Nonstress testing should begin at 26 weeks and continue until delivery. The length of time between tests is determined by the severity of renal disease and hypertension. It should be done at least once a week starting at 26 weeks and twice a week starting at 32 weeks.
- Fetal growth ultrasonographic measurements should be taken at 26, 32, and 36 weeks. In terms of growth, the amniotic fluid index (AFI), baby weight, and gestation age should all be considered. Doppler studies may be required as well.
- The biophysical profile adds to the picture of the fetal state. It should be done at the same time as nonstress testing and at similar intervals.

DELIVERY

- Pregnancy can be safely extended until term if blood pressure is adequately controlled, renal function is not deteriorating, and fetal growth and well-being are satisfactory.
- In the absence of premature delivery or of fetal distress, vaginal delivery should be considered.
- Women at higher risk of volume depletion or fluid overload should be identified prior to birth so that their fluid status can be monitored before intravenous fluids are provided.
- The aim of this supervision is to ensure euvolemia and the avoidance of both pulmonary edema and superimposed kidney injury.
- Fluid balance testing should be performed by a qualified clinician who is familiar with the hemodynamic changes that occur throughout pregnancy and the puerperium.

POSTPARTUM

- Short-term nonsteroidal anti-inflammatory medication side effects in people without preexisting risk factors are thought to be uncommon.
- In the postpartum period, nonsteroidal anti-inflammatory drugs (NSAIDs) are currently indicated for perineal pain when paracetamol is insufficient to relieve symptoms.
- During pregnancy, women with known or newly discovered renal illness should continue to see their nephrologist.
- They should be offered early contraceptive advice in the form of progesterone only-pill, a progesterone subdermal implant, and the progesterone intrauterine system.
- Women who use prednisolone, hydroxychloroquine, azathioprine, cyclosporine, tacrolimus, enalapril, captopril, amlodipine, nifedipine, labetalol, atenolol, and low molecular weight heparin can nurse their babies.
- Postnatal evaluation of women with early-onset preeclampsia is important to identify women with underlying renal disease.
- If isolated microscopic hematuria with structurally normal kidneys persists after delivery and has not been treated during pregnancy, it should be investigated.
- For lifelong follow-up and monitoring, women with renal disease require a multidisciplinary team.

CONCLUSION

Renal disease is relatively common in young women and may be caused by a variety of underlying conditions. Prepregnancy counseling to optimize care prior to pregnancy and careful multi-disciplinary team approach are key to providing the best outcomes.

SUGGESTED READING

1. Gonzalez Suarez ML, Kattah A, Grande JP, Garovic V. Renal Disorders in Pregnancy: Core Curriculum 2019. Am J Kidney Dis. 2019;73(1):119-30.
2. Hladunewich MA, Melamed N, Bramham K. Pregnancy across the spectrum of chronic kidney disease. Kidney Int. 2016;89(5):995-1007.
3. Wiles K, Chappell L, Clark K, Elman L, Hall M, Lightstone L, et al. Clinical practice guideline on pregnancy and renal disease. BMC Nephrol. 2019;20:401.

11

CHAPTER

Dialysis in Pregnancy

INTRODUCTION

Despite reduced fertility in women with advanced chronic kidney disease (CKD) undergoing dialysis, pregnancies still occur. Dialysis has improved outcomes and successful birth rates have risen to 70–90%.

Complications associated with dialysis are:
- Hypertension (50–70%)
- Preeclampsia (18–67%)
- Polyhydramnios (40%)
- Intrauterine growth restriction (17–77%)
- Placental abruption
- Blood transfusions
- Prematurity and low birth weight (50–100%)

The indications for acute dialysis during pregnancy are:
- Severe refractory metabolic acidosis
- Electrolyte imbalance, especially severe refractory hyperkalemia
- Volume overload leading to congestive heart failure
- Pulmonary edema that is unresponsive to diuretics
- Maternal urea concentration is >17 mmol/L.

Because of the higher risk of fetal death, dialysis may be started earlier in pregnancy if there is an abrupt worsening in renal function.

PRECONCEPTION

- During pregnancy, a multidisciplinary team of obstetricians, nephrologist, anesthetists, and physicians are needed with a well-equipped dialysis center.
- Residual renal function is an important indicator contributing to improved pregnancy outcomes in women starting dialysis.
- Women who are on dialysis before pregnancy should be counseled about the possibility of deferring pregnancy until transplantation (if possible) and the requirement for extended, frequent dialysis prior to and during pregnancy.
- Women receiving hemodialysis during pregnancy should aim for a predialysis urea of < 12.5 mmol/L and women on peritoneal dialysis prior to pregnancy should be converted to hemodialysis.

ANTENATAL

Aim

- Predialysis blood urea nitrogen (BUN) <50 mg/dL (17.9 mmol/L) or
- Urea <100 mg/dL (16.6 mmol/L)

Dialysis

- A gentle start (e.g., 2 hours, three times per week) with titration according to biochemical parameters and maternal-fetal wellbeing should be initiated. Weekly hemodialysis is gradually raised from 12 to 20 hours, and a high-efficacy dialyzer with a biocompatible membrane is utilized.
- The blood flow is maintained from 180 to 240 mL/min at an average and the dialysate flow at 500 mL/min. Low-molecular-weight heparin (LMWH) 1,000 IU bolus dose followed by 250 IU every hour is given to minimize the hemorrhagic risk and to avoid coagulation of the dialyzer as shown in **Figure 1**.
- Weekly hemodialysis hours are determined by urine output (1 L), time on dialysis prior to pregnancy (1 year), and weight (70 kg), and then adjusted based on midweek predialysis serum urea, blood pressure, weight gain, polyhydramnios, and uremic symptoms.

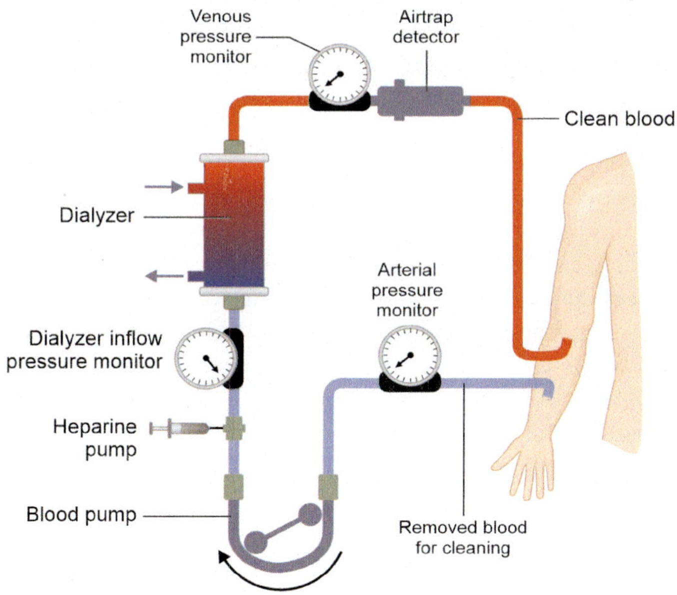

Fig. 1: Mechanism of dialysis.
Source: https://www.google.com/url?sa=i&url=https%3A%2F%2Fwww.researchgate.net%2Ffigure%2FSchematic-visualization-of-a-hemodialysis-circuit_fig2_281733078&psig=AOvVaw1k1bGVUzuAJqqEgrLoyhOv&ust=1734610072750000&source=images&cd=vfe&opi=89978449&ved=0CBcQjhxqFwoTCOCp5-CisYoDFQAAAAAdAAAAABAE

- Long-hours dialysis achieves lower maternal urea levels, reduced fetal-osmotic diuresis and polyhydramnios. It avoids rapid fluid shifts, uteroplacental hypoperfusion, and fetal distress.
- Dry weight is controlled by slow continuous ultrafiltration to achieve the goal of 0.5 kg on weight gain per week.

Blood Pressure

- Maintain blood pressure level < 140/90 mm Hg as explained in **Table 1**.
- To avoid mid-dialysis hypotension (<120/70 mm Hg), the pregnant women should be treated by combination of ultrafiltration assessments and blood pressure drugs, such as calcium antagonist and alpha-methyldopa.

Diet

- It should be unrestricted and rich in protein (1.5–1.8 g/kg IBW/day).
- Calorie intake of 35–40 kcal/kg/day.
- Calcitriol and calcium carbonate of 0.25 μg/day and 0.6 g/day.

Electrolytes

- Magnesium, potassium, and calcium-phosphate balance should be monitored every 1–2 weeks and supplementation maybe needed.
- *Vitamin supplementation*: Folic acid and water-soluble vitamins lost during dialysis must be taken into account, with supplementation as indicated, including high-dose folic acid (5 mg) prepregnancy and during the first trimester.

Anemia

- Patients should get 10,000 IU of subcutaneous recombinant human erythropoietin twice a week. Supplementing with intravenous iron sucrose at a rate of 100 mg biweekly and 10 mg folic acid is recommended.
- Lower conception rates in women receiving peritoneal dialysis have been reported. Hypertonic fluid and adhesions disturbing implantation are responsible. In case of vascular access problems, logistical impediments to frequent hemodialysis, and good residual renal function, continuing peritoneal dialysis may be considered.

DELIVERY

- The delivery should be scheduled at a facility that has the resources to handle complicated maternal and fetal circumstances.
- Administration of magnesium sulfate for impending eclampsia or fetal neuroprotection in cases of preterm delivery should be done with caution.
- Induction of labor is considered at 37–39 weeks of gestation to avoid spontaneous labor in an anticoagulated woman.
- Vaginal delivery should be considered unless an obstetric indication for lower segment caesarean section.

TABLE 1: Management of pregnancy in women on dialysis.

<table>
<tr><th>Preconception</th><th>First trimester (weeks 0–13)</th><th>Second trimester (weeks 14–27)</th><th>Third trimester (weeks 28–40)</th><th>Delivery</th><th>Postpartum</th></tr>
<tr><td rowspan="3">• Discuss family planning including timing. outcomes, transplant
• Review medications and stop those that are potentially teratogenic
• Optimize comorbid conditions (diabetes, lupus, obesity, etc.)
• Monthly serum pregnancy test if irregular menses
• Establish multidisciplinary care (nephrology, high-risk obstetrics)</td><td colspan="3">• Intensify hemodialysis (36 hours/week or BUN < 35 mg/dL)
• q2 week labs, adjust dialysate, ESA, iron as needed
• Blood pressure target <140/90 or DBP 85 mm Hg; avoid hypotension <120/70 mm Hg
• ASA 75–150 mg daily, folic acid 5 mg daily, liberalize diet</td><td rowspan="3">• Plan induction at or around 37 weeks
• Ensure neonatal services available including intensive care
• Heparin-free dialysis to allow for use of epidural
• If needed for preeclampsia, reduce Mg dose by 50%, monitor levels at least every 4 hours
• Vaginal delivery preferred; typical obstetric indications for caesarean delivery</td><td rowspan="3">• Support breastfeeding if desired; review medications for lactation safety and avoid iatrogenic hypovolemia
• Can resume prepregnancy hemodialysis regimen
• Monitor for signs of postpartum depression and ensure adequate social support
• Provide appropriate contraception</td></tr>
<tr><td rowspan="2">• Ultrasound to establish intrauterine pregnancy and accurate gestational age
• First trimester screen for aneuploidy</td><td colspan="2">• Adjust EDW for anticipated 0.3–0.5 kg/week weight gain
• Starting at 22–26 weeks; q2 week BPP, fetal growth, umbilical artery Doppler, preeclampsia labs including LFTs</td></tr>
<tr><td>• 20 weeks ultrasound for fetal anomalies, cervical length
• 22 weeks placental ultrasound with Doppler</td><td>Increase frequency of fetal monitoring to weekly; earlier if needed for complications</td></tr>
</table>

(ASA: aspirin; BPP: biophysical profile; BUN: blood urea nitrogen; DBP: diastolic blood pressure; EDW: estimated dry weight; ESA: erythropoiesis-stimulating agent; LFTs: liver function tests; Mg: magnesium)

Source: Oliverio AL, Hladunewich MA. End-Stage Kidney Disease and Dialysis in Pregnancy. Adv Chronic Kidney Dis. 2020;27(6):477-485.

POSTPARTUM

- Breastfeeding is safe in women undergoing dialysis.
- Providers also should be attentive to avoid overaggressive ultrafiltration and dehydration, which might impede breast milk supply.
- Patient can resume prepregnancy hemodialysis regime as explained in **Table 1**.
- Check for postpartum depression and counsel for an effective method of contraception.

CONCLUSION

Successful pregnancy is possible in women of childbearing age under replacement therapy for kidney function. In the last decades, the dialysis treatment optimization has helped increase the rate of live births; however, these pregnancies have a higher risk of fetal and maternal complications when compared to pregnancies of women who are not on dialysis.

Today, we know that hemodialysis and peritoneal dialysis can be replacement therapy options. Main measures to be taken include increasing the weekly dialysis time, maintaining low levels of predialysis urea, controlling anemia and preventing infections, tension and electrolytic oscillations. To ensure best outcomes, the multidisciplinary care provided by nephrologists, obstetricians, pediatricians, nutritionists and psychologists is becoming increasingly important.

SUGGESTED READING

1. Bode AS, Tordoir J. Vascular Access for Hemodialysis Therapy. Stud Comput Intell. 2013;404:235-303.
2. Oliverio AL, Hladunewich MA. End-Stage Kidney Disease and Dialysis in Pregnancy. Adv Chronic Kidney Dis. 2020;27(6):477-85.
3. Ribeiro CI, Silva N. Pregnancy and dialysis. J Bras Nefrol. 2020;42(3):349-56.
4. Wiles K, Chappell L, Clark K, Elman L, Hall M, Lightstone L, et al. Clinical practice guideline on pregnancy and renal disease. BMC Nephrol. 2019;20:401.

CHAPTER 12

Multiple Choice Questions

1. **A common marker of chronic kidney disease (CKD) is:**
   a. Rash
   b. Hematuria
   c. Proteinuria
   d. Bacteremia

Ans. c. Proteinuria

2. **The two leading causes of end-stage renal disease (ESRD) are:**
   a. Allergies and diabetes
   b. Infection and diabetes
   c. Diabetes and hypertension
   d. Infection and hypertension

Ans. c. Diabetes and hypertension

3. **The leading genetic cause of ESRD in the United States is:**
   a. Diabetes
   b. Alport syndrome
   c. Autosomal recessive polycystic kidney disease
   d. Autosomal dominant polycystic kidney disease

Ans. d. Autosomal dominant polycystic kidney disease

4. **Acute kidney injury (AKI) rates are significantly associated with aging and with:**
   a. White race
   b. Low income
   c. Female sex
   d. Body mass index (BMI)

Ans. d. Body mass index (BMI)

5. **The most common type of AKI according to pathophysiology is:**
   a. Diabetic
   b. Prerenal
   c. Postrenal
   d. Intrarenal

Ans. b. Prerenal

6. **Suspicion for mild renal disease should be based on:**
   a. The presence of proteinuria
   b. Clinical signs and symptoms
   c. Patient physical examination
   d. Recognition of the primary pathologic mechanism responsible for renal injury

Ans. d. Recognition of the primary pathologic mechanism responsible for renal injury

7. The most important tool in monitoring patients with suspected and diagnosed renal failure is:

a. Dipstick urinalysis
b. Kidney ultrasound
c. Auscultation of lung sounds
d. Serum creatinine measurements

Ans. a. Dipstick urinalysis

8. Intrarenal AKI may be recognized by a distinctive presentation of:

a. Orthostatic hypotension
b. Edema of the extremities
c. Very high urine osmolality
d. Brownish, muddy appearance of urine

Ans. c. Very high urine osmolality

9. Which of the following factors indicates an increased risk of advancement to higher stages of kidney disease?

a. Proteinuria
b. Increasing glomerular filtration rate (GFR)
c. Older age at diagnosis
d. Hematuria of nonrenal origin

Ans. a. Proteinuria

10. For patients with stage 1 or 2 renal disease, cardiovascular risk should be assessed:

a. Monthly
b. Every 6 months
c. Annually
d. Every 2 years

Ans. c. Annually

11. The leading cause of death among patients with ESRD is:

a. Uremia
b. Anemia
c. Liver failure
d. Cardiovascular complications

Ans. d. Cardiovascular complications

12. The use of angiotensin-converting enzyme (ACE) inhibitors has been shown to be beneficial in patients with:

a. Lupus
b. Hypotension
c. Renal artery stenosis
d. Diabetic nephropathy

Ans. d. Diabetic nephropathy

13. Patients with diabetes and CKD should have a low-density lipoprotein (LDL) goal of less than:

a. 50 mg/dL
b. 70 mg/dL
c. 100 mg/dL
d. 130 mg/dL

Ans. b. 70 mg/dL

14. Patients with CKD should limit daily phosphorus intake to:

a. 0.8–1.2 g
b. 3–5 g
c. 8–12 g
d. <60 g

Ans. a. 0.8–1.2 g

15. Which of the following medications require dosage adjustment in patients with renal failure?

a. Digoxin
b. Opioids
c. Antifungals
d. All of the above

Ans. d. All of the above

16. Stage 4 CKD may require the use of exogenous erythropoietin to manage:

a. Anemia
b. Neutropenia
c. Pancytopenia
d. Thrombocytopenia

Ans. a. Anemia

17. ESRD is commonly defined as a GFR less than:

a. 15 mL/min/1.73 m^2
b. 25 mL/min/1.73 m^2
c. 35 mL/min/1.73 m^2
d. 45 mL/min/1.73 m^2

Ans. a.15 mL/min/1.73 m^2

18. For adults with ESRD who are receiving hemodialysis, the recommended maximum daily intake of protein is:

a. 0.1–0.4 g/kg
b. 0.6–0.8 g/kg
c. 1.1–1.4 g/kg
d. 11–14 g/kg

Ans. c. 1.1–1.4 g/kg

19. Hemodialysis can be provided via:

a. Arteriovenous graft
b. Arteriovenous fistula
c. Temporary venous catheter
d. All of the above

Ans. d. All of the above

20. Patency of the arteriovenous fistula can be assessed by:

a. Palpating a thrill
b. Auscultating a bruit
c. Taking a blood pressure of the fistula
d. Both a and b

Ans. d. Both a and b

21. Which of the following is a contraindication to renal transplantation?

a. Hypertension
b. human immunodeficiency virus (HIV) infection
c. Metastatic cancer
d. Age older than 50 years

Ans. c. Metastatic cancer

22. In the United States, the median adult wait time for a cadaver kidney is:

a. 1 year
b. 2.3 years
c. 4 years
d. 10.6 years

Ans. c. 4 years

23. Which of the following has been shown to help prevent contrast-induced nephropathy in patients with CKD?

a. Mannitol
b. Furosemide
c. ACE inhibitors
d. Sodium bicarbonate infusion

Ans. d. Sodium bicarbonate infusion

24. The most common form of renal disease in patients with HIV is:

a. Nephropathy
b. Preeclampsia
c. Lupus nephritis
d. Glomerulonephritis

Ans. a. Nephropathy

25. In a typical, uncomplicated pregnancy, which of the following renal changes occur?

a. Increased GFR
b. Decreased kidney size
c. Decreased renal plasma flow
d. Fewer urinary tract infections

Ans. a. Increased GFR

26. Preeclampsia is a syndrome of:

a. Late-term seizures
b. Hypotension and hematuria
c. Hypertension and proteinuria
d. Hyperglycemia and hemorrhage

Ans. c. Hypertension and proteinuria

27. In pregnancies after renal transplantation, fetal survival rates are:

a. 25%
b. 50%
c. 75%
d. 90%

Ans. d. 90%

28. When prescribing selective serotonin reuptake inhibitors to patients with CKD, the dose should:

a. Be increased
b. Be decreased
c. Remain the same

d. Be adjusted according to renal clearance

Ans. c. Remain the same

29. Chronic illness can be the source of ambiguous loss, which is defined as loss:

a. Of sense of self
b. Without accompanying grief, sorrow, or mourning
c. Experienced by those with no close relationship to the patient
d. Without the finality of death but also with no certainty of returning to previous levels of functioning

Ans. d. Without the finality of death but also with no certainty of returning to previous levels of functioning

30. Hospice is generally approved for patients with ESRD who:

a. Are candidates for dialysis
b. Have a serum creatinine level <15 mg/dL
c. Have a creatinine clearance <15 mL/minute
d. All of the above

Ans. c. Have a creatinine clearance <15 mL/minute

Index

Page numbers followed by *b* refer to box *f* refer to figure, *fc* refer to flowchart and *t* refer to table

L

M

N

O

P

Q

R

S

T

U

V